CW00708674

Joy Melville is a full-time writer and author of *Phobias and Obsessions* (Optima), *The Tranquillizer Trap* (Fontana), *The ABC of Eating* (Sheldon Press) and *First Aid in Mental Health* (Allen & Unwin).

Dr Fiona Subotsky is a Consultant Child Psychiatrist at King's College Hospital in London. She has worked with unhappy children and their families for the last 15 years in a variety of different settings, and became aware that parents might be helped even before approaching a service such as child guidance if they knew a little more about it. She has two children of her own, now grown up.

Phyllis S.

Does My Child Need Help?

A Guide for Worried Parents

JOY MELVILLE
and
DR FIONA SUBOTSKY

An OPTIMA book

Copyright © Joy Melville and Dr Fiona Subotsky, 1992

First published in Great Britain in 1992 by Optima,
a division of Little, Brown and Company (UK) Limited.

A CIP catalogue record for this book
is available from the British Library.

Typeset by Leaper & Gard Ltd, Bristol
Printed in England by Clays Ltd, St Ives plc

ISBN 0 356 20979 2

Little, Brown and Company (UK) Limited
165 Great Dover Street
London SE1 4YA

CONTENTS

INTRODUCTION

'How long do you expect your child to attend the clinic?' parents were asked in a questionnaire prepared by a child guidance clinic. The replies ranged from 'Not too long' to 'A year' to 'No idea'.

'Which professionals do you expect to see?' was another question. Again, replies varied widely: 'Child psychologist'; 'Social worker'; 'Psychiatric social worker'; 'Someone in the medical profession'; 'Child guidance counsellor'; 'Doctor'; and 'Not sure'.

Replies to these questions highlighted parents' widespread bewilderment and lack of knowledge about what to expect when taking their child for therapy. The purpose of this book is to help dispel such ignorance and to act as a practical guide to parents.

Many parents do not know how to assess the seriousness of their child's abnormal behaviour in the first place. Is their child seriously withdrawn, for instance, or simply going through a bad phase? How can they tell whether the behaviour is temporary and unimportant or needs skilled help?

Where, too, do they go for help? Their GP? A private psychiatrist? A child guidance clinic? Or the teacher at school? Who will be the professional who sees their child? How often? Will they be able to be there themselves? Will

they have to fill out a lot of forms? Will these be confidential? What actually happens when they take their
child for treatment? If it is suggested that the whole family
participate in family therapy, what will that entail?

Because there is still a stigma surrounding psychological or psychiatric treatment of any kind, parents of
children whose behaviour is, or appears to be, abnormal in
some way remain reticent, even secretive about it. They do
not casually chat about the problems or seek advice from
relatives, neighbours or other parents they happen to meet
at the school gates. There are rarely 'parent guidance'
classes, like ante-natal classes, that they could attend and
learn what to do in a crisis situation.

As a result, parents don't have the opportunity to
compare their children's behaviour and may worry about a
minor problem or ignore a major one. Lone parents, in
particular, may not have anyone with whom they may
discuss their concerns.

The reasons given by parents for bringing their child to
the child guidance clinic reveal some of the most common
concerns. One parent, asked her reason for coming,
possibly summed it all up when she answered with two
words: 'My son'.

Others gave a little more detail, with behaviour being
frequently mentioned: 'To find out why my child's behaviour is deteriorating,' said one parent. 'Because of a
complaint from school about my child's behaviour,' said
another. Many mentioned general behaviour problems.
One child wouldn't go outside the flat, for instance; one
son consistently stayed out late; another child refused to
go to school but rejected any help. Other problems
included the child having nightmares; creating problems
at home and at school; being generally troublesome;
wetting or soiling the bed and having a difficult attitude.

A century ago, parental discipline was very strict and

parents expected to have complete control over their children. The upbringing and education of middle- and upper-class children was largely in the hands of nannies and governesses; while working-class children were often sent out to work at a very young age.

Nowadays the wheel has turned full circle. Many parents feel they no longer have any control over their children and are unable to cope with their behaviour. They feel they need help, even if they are not sure where to turn.

The variation in the kind of help parents wanted was evident from the replies given in the child guidance survey to the question: 'What do you hope to change or achieve by coming to the clinic?' Some treated the clinic as a sort of Citizens' Advice Bureau, wanting information about playgroups and suggestions about what the child should play. But most parents had come because of more specific concerns about their child's conduct. Some children were showing obvious signs of distress. They were withdrawn, for instance, or constantly soiling, or behaving oddly. Parents were anxious to know whether their child had any psychological problems and wanted help to understand or to change their child's disruptive or defiant behaviour, which was frequently affecting the mood of the entire family.

One parent wanted 'To improve my son's behaviour and make him realise wrong from right.' 'I'd like a better idea of how I can deal with the problems bothering my child,' said another – a sentiment that was endorsed by a number of parents. 'To change my son's attitude and his aggressiveness' and 'To sort his behaviour out so that I can get to know him better' were typical of further hopes and wishes.

There was concern about the unhappiness of a son or daughter – 'Could you make my daughter feel better about herself?'; 'Could you help my son not to be scared of the outside?'; 'Could you find out why he wakes up crying at night?' Sometimes the parent knew that the child's behaviour was caused by problems at school, but still did not know how to handle the situation.

This book cannot cure a child's difficult behaviour. But what it will do is to alert parents to the warning signs of distress and disturbance and demystify what happens when parents and children see a psychiatrist or psychologist, attend a child guidance clinic, or take part in family therapy.

1

SHOULD I WORRY ABOUT THIS?

Children do and say surprising things. Often parents wonder whether, for instance, an incident of stealing or a relapse into bed-wetting is something to worry about or even a reason to take the child to the doctor. This chapter comprises an alphabetical list of symptoms and problems, with some advice on how to think about them and what to do.

AGGRESSIVENESS

Aggressiveness is one of those words often used which needs to be 'unpacked'. What does the teacher mean exactly if she says your child is aggressive at school? Is this hitting other boys or girls of his or her own age, getting into tempers, bullying smaller children, swearing at the teacher or teasing the class guinea-pig? Or all of these? How often do these incidents occur? What precedes them? What follows them? Can some adults seem to deal with them better than others? Do many of the other children behave in the same way? What are the school's policies for dealing with such behaviour? Some parents disagree with the school on whether their child should be expected to fight back or not, and this will need sorting out.

Asking similar questions about 'aggressiveness' at home can also be illuminating and may generate ideas as to how to better cope with the problem – if such it is. Think not only what might possibly be upsetting your child to cause behaviour like this, but from where he or she may be learning it.

Children are great imitators and there are many possible models these days, from television and videos to actually witnessing or experiencing violence in the home.

Girls are less often described as aggressive than boys. When this does occur it is sometimes not much more than 'unladylike' boisterousness that might pass completely unnoticed in a boy and actually be a useful quality in later life. With both boys and girls energy and assertiveness are the plus sides of 'aggressiveness' and need channelling in more socially constructive ways.

ANXIETY

Anxiety, fearfulness and worrying happen in everyone's life from time to time and can often be used constructively to think through how to cope with, and master, some future event which seems difficult or uncertain. So trying to prevent children from having any worries at all may not be the best way to help them cope with the demands of growing up and adult life. Indeed, if the only signs of disturbance are those of worry, some doctors would rate this of comparatively little significance, and likely to pass. However, if a child shows great anxiety this certainly means that they are in current distress and is a sign that they are having to deal with some stress which is too much for them at their particular stage of emotional development.

It may be obvious to you as the parent what this might

be – for instance a three-year-old who has just come out of hospital might be more than usually clinging. In this kind of situation, meeting the child's need for extra attention and reassurance of security (allowing your child into your bed temporarily for instance) may be all that is necessary.

Sometimes, you may know quite well the source of stress – for example, that you and your partner have been arguing a great deal – but not be able to put this right by yourself. And sometimes, you may not know the cause of the problem at all. In the last two types of cases, it is sensible to ask for help, whether from family and friends or professionals.

APPETITE AND WEIGHT LOSS

Children, like adults, may lose their appetites during and after an episode of illness or severe worry. Unlike adults, however, the responsibility for feeding children lies with their parents, and so the mismatch of the child's appetite and the parents' wish to feed the child may cause considerable conflict at meal times. Sometimes things become so bad, especially with young children who have never 'fed well' or who were perhaps in hospital and dependent on tube feeding, that it becomes a battle of wills with much unhappiness created all round. (See also Failure to Thrive below.)

If appetite loss persists, especially if there is weight loss, do seek the advice of your GP as there are many reasons, often physical, why this might occur. However, if you then hear the word 'anorexia' used, bear in mind in strict medical terms it only means absence or loss of appetite, so do not assume that your child has the much more serious condition of anorexia nervosa. (See also the section on anorexia nervosa in Chapter 5.)

BED-WETTING

Bed-wetting, or enuresis in the medical terminology, is obviously completely normal for babies and toddlers. While day-time dryness is usually achieved around the age of two to three, and night-time dryness a bit later, there are considerable individual variations. Often there are periods when a child lapses back into more immature behaviour and these can have both psychological and physical causes.

Bear in mind that 10–15 per cent of five-year-olds still wet their beds sometimes, and most will simply grow out of this in time. Nevertheless, it can be very embarrassing for the child and quite a strain on the family's patience.

Your GP, health visitor, school nurse or school doctor can advise. There may be special clinics run locally which can undertake any necessary physical investigations and advise on management. Often a star chart is suggested first to encourage dryness, and this can be especially helpful in promoting a more positive approach. Wetting alarms can also be very useful and the models available are improving. Parents may have to put in quite a lot of effort with this method as the alarms first have to be set up in the bedding and on the child, and when the alarm goes off the parent has to take the child to the toilet and reset the alarm. Children over the age of 10 or 11 may be able to manage the newer kinds of alarm themselves as these are less bulky.

For persistent bed-wetting, medicines are sometimes prescribed and are effective with some children, though relapse is common after the medicine is stopped. A nasal spray is now available on prescription which, it is claimed, reduces night wetting. It is a fairly new product and may prove useful.

Some children seem to wet the bed as part of a general

pattern of emotional disturbance and for these referral to a child guidance clinic is best.

BITING

Biting is an unpleasant but common behaviour usually found in the under-fives. It is best not to over-react – and certainly to resist the temptation to bite back – even if you or a younger sibling were the victim. However, make it clear that biting is not acceptable, and hopefully it will be a phase that will pass rapidly.

BOREDOM

Asking your child for the reason for a particular misdemeanour often leads to one of the two classic responses 'I dunno' and 'I was bored'. Children these days tend to have a short attention span which is reinforced by high-impact, high-speed computer games and TV shows. Giving them more and more of this type of entertainment is unlikely to help, so encourage any sign you may see of a more creative or social interest from stamp collecting to swimming, where the individual effort put in is clearly part of the fun. Be prepared for your child not only to share in some of your interests, but also to differ sometimes too. For instance, was it you or your children who really wanted that computer, train set, outing or satellite dish?

BULLYING

If your child is accused of being a bully at school this may be a cause for serious concern, and may be quite difficult

to deal with. As you try and find out what is going on, you
will need all your patience not to feel either the school or
your child is completely in the wrong. An outside professional's help or advice can often be very useful in this kind
of situation. (See also Chapter 7.)

CRUELTY TO ANIMALS

Even a one-off incident of cruelty to animals should be
taken very seriously as a sign of a more deep-rooted
disturbance, especially if it is carried out by a child on his
or her own rather than in a badly-behaving group or gang.
It would be very appropriate, especially if there are other
signs of difficulties, to insist that your child is referred to a
child guidance clinic.

DAY-DREAMING

Parents are rightly not usually worried if their child is said
by others to be 'a bit of a dreamer'. Day-dreaming as a
happy preoccupation and an escape from the maths lesson
could even have its uses in later life. Some parents,
however, become concerned that their child 'seems to be
in a trance' and even wonder if this is some kind of
epileptic fit. Usually this is not the case but it is quite
reasonable to ask that a child behaving in this way should
be checked by a paediatrician. Day-dreaming can also
consist of unhappy or distressing thoughts – a bit like
nightmares during the day. Children can sometimes be
upset by this sort of worrying and describe them as 'bad
thoughts' and even wonder if they are going mad. Get
advice as this sort of problem can usually be helped, sometimes quite simply, and is most unlikely to be a form of
real mental illness.

DEFIANCE AND DISOBEDIENCE

Parents do not want a robot for a child, so rarely demand complete unquestioning obedience on all occasions. On the other hand if you cannot get your child to refrain from dangerous or anti-social behaviour, or to do the things which you consider important, such as helping in the house, problems may build up for the future. Some parents may be observed unconsciously training their child to disobey – for instance, telling a small child not to touch something but not intervening as well. Occasional subsequent punishment, even if apparently well-deserved, often does not reduce the unwanted behaviour. If you find your reasonable demands defied or ignored by a young child, take your time and for a while only issue orders which you can actually enforce gently but firmly. For older children, again limit your requests – don't nag – and be pleased by any positive responses. But remember that mothers and fathers have rights too, particularly not to be insulted.

Beware of the classic situation where the child won't do what one adult asks, but runs to complain to another if the first tells him off. This commonly happens between mother and father, but also between parent and school and can easily lead to a row breaking out between the adults while the child continues on his own way.

DRINKING

There is evidence that children who see their parents drinking alcohol in moderation at home and even sometimes take part in it are at less risk of alcohol problems later than children who come from homes where there is total abstention or where alcohol is taken to excess. Children also like to experiment and imitate adult ways, so a 'one-off' trial of the sherry may be only a passing nuisance.

But there are additional risks for teenagers in the greater availability of alcohol outside the home, such as at uncritical pubs or cans from supermarkets. Groups of teenagers drinking excessively together may not only be an irritation to more sober citizens but can also become involved in serious risk-taking behaviour because alcohol lowers inhibitions. They may also be setting up a pattern of behaviour which will harm their health and social relationships later. If a young teenager is drinking alcohol alone this is even more serious and help should certainly be sought. (The organisation Alanon may be useful to contact – see Useful Addresses on page 226.)

DRUG-TAKING

Parents have different views on their children using drugs as they do with alcohol. Warnings are unfortunately as likely to encourage curious experimentation as to put children off, but prevention is certainly easier than cure. Without constant questioning try to ensure that you know where your teenager is, who with, and doing what. Setting limits of this type may provoke some argument at first, but is usually secretly respected by the teenager as a mark of caring. If you begin to have serious worries about possible drug abuse, do ask other parents and at the school to see if there is known to be a group problem of some kind. Professionals such as GPs may not be well-informed simply because this kind of behaviour is not usually brought to their attention. (See also Chapter 5.)

ENURESIS

See bed-wetting.

EXPOSURE

In recent years, when child sexual abuse has been so much in the news, it has become very difficult to evaluate what is normal or abnormal about a young child's sexual behaviour. However, an experienced infant or nursery teacher will have seen all sorts of behaviour in the Wendy House over many years and will be well placed to judge how to react if two five-year-olds decide to show each other their genitals. If the behaviour is repeated, or anxiety-associated, then there will be cause for concern. If your child is involved it may well be best if you take the initiative and ask for professional assessment and help, for instance through your GP.

'FAILURE TO THRIVE'

You may hear this expression used of a baby or toddler who is not putting on weight at anything like the normal rate. After the health visitor, clinic doctor and GP have made their assessments, if progress continues to be un-satisfactory then the child may be seen by a hospital paediatrician for detailed physical investigations. If these also prove negative then social and psychological factors are also considered.

This is intended to be helpful but may sometimes be seen as threatening by parents, especially if a social worker or child psychiatrist is called in and there are questions about whether the child is 'at risk' of neglect or emotional abuse. Because some parents do, often unintentionally, harm their children's development, these processes are necessary, but can obviously be an additional source of great anxiety. The mental health professionals are usually very aware of this and should be more keen to find out what they can do to help than to make open or implied accusations. If you get involved in such a situation try to establish a continuing relationship with a professional whom you respect and trust, as whatever the reason for it, this type of problem often needs a lot of effort to overcome.

FEARS

Children's fears are common and various – from the cracks in the pavement to the noise of the wind at night. These will increase at times of stress and insecurity and especially if the child has actually undergone some recent unpleasant experience such as witnessing a road accident or being the victim of a mugging. Let your child tell you about his or her fears without rushing – even if it is something totally fanciful like monsters or witches under the bed. Usually such fears pass as the stress is coped with, but if they persist or are particularly distressing then help should be sought.

Some possibilities for prevention include monitoring what younger children see on television – news of war and disasters can be as frightening as horror films – and not making over-alarming threats such as 'If you do that again you'll give Daddy a heart attack'.

FIGHTING

It is not abnormal for children to fight, but if you are being driven mad by your children fighting at home what can you do? Typically parents of three children will say 'Any two are fine but ...' and parents of two children will say 'Either of them alone is fine but ...'. Or parents may be convinced that only one of the children – usually the older one – is to blame. He or she, of course, claims it is always started by the younger one.

This is not an easy suggestion but try not to get sucked into asking for detailed histories of the incident or taking sides. If the younger one knows you are not going to intervene, for instance, the motivation for increasing the volume of screams will suddenly diminish. Make a rule about fighting only taking place outside or upstairs. Make sure the adults stick together and are consistent with the rules and any penalties. If your best efforts are unsuccessful, and the situation is really upsetting family life, family therapy can often help with this problem. (See also Aggressiveness.)

FIRE-STARTING

Fires are exciting and attractive, partly because of their capacity to be unpredictably dangerous. Many small boys have severely damaged their homes when experiments with matches have got out of control. A continued preoccupation with fires and matches may be a sign of disturbance and is sometimes combined with setting off fire alarms or calling out the fire brigade. With a seriously emotionally disturbed child this can merely be the most dangerous of many other symptoms of disturbance. If the fire-starting is repeated, get help.

GLUE-SNIFFING

Glues and other solvents are attractive to children as they can give a 'high' or a 'buzz' and are more easily available than alcohol or other drugs. Glue-sniffing is usually a group activity found in rather disaffected and unsupervised teenage boys and sometimes girls, and can just be part of a phase. However, there can be serious physical consequences, both directly from the chemicals in the solvent and from dangerous behaviour that may follow due to the alteration of consciousness. In addition, a pattern of trying to blank out depression and boredom in this way may lead to greater problems later. Do your best to intervene and ensure safety by supervision; threats and warnings are not usually successful. (See also drinking and drug-taking.)

Re-solv is a helpful organisation to contact (see Useful Addresses on page 238).

GRAFFITI

Adolescents who become involved with writing graffiti, as with other forms of excitingly risky but anti-social behaviour, seem rarely to be brought to the attention of child mental health professionals by their parents, GPs or schools. Presumably they have already become skilled avoiders of unwanted adult attention, and there is the common dilemma for parents of not knowing whether it is best to ignore the situation and hope it will go away, or to intervene heavily. However, graffiti writing is sometimes undertaken in dangerous situations, such as the Underground, so it should be prevented by parents if possible. You may need to consider whether further help is needed by your offspring or your family; as well as considering other aspects of your offspring's adjustment and personality before deciding on the right approach.

HAIR-PULLING

It is quite common, though it is often not noticed, for children to go through a phase of pulling out their own hair. It seems to be the sort of 'nervous habit' which provides a temporary reduction of anxiety, so parental intervention which increases anxiety such as telling the child off is likely to make matters worse. If the underlying stress and tension is considerable then help may be needed to overcome that.

HEAD-BANGING

Babies often go through a phase of banging their heads against the side of the cot as part of a rocking movement, and sometimes this persists into toddlerhood. Usually there are no ill-effects apart from the noise. If any harm is coming to the child, however, and handicapped children do sometimes damage themselves in this way, then help should be sought from a specialist.

HEARING VOICES

Children sometimes say that they hear a voice telling them to do something, for instance steal some sweets, and are unclear whether this is coming from outside their head or from inside. In case there are associated worries, it is sensible to listen closely to what the child is saying about this – perhaps he or she is afraid to 'own' the wish or deed themselves. But don't panic: this kind of experience has been shown to be more common with both adults and children than had previously been realised.

HYPERACTIVITY

Perhaps as many as 50 per cent of parents of young boys think their son is 'overactive', so you are not alone if you have this concern. It may or may not be helpful to consider this kind of behaviour as a kind of disease, but there is no doubt it is wearing on parents' nerves. For further information see Chapter 5.

JEALOUSY

Jealousy, particularly of a younger brother or sister, is an extremely common cause of childhood misbehaviour and consequent family tension. This can happen even and perhaps especially in the most loving of families.

Jealousy can also be evident in a child's attitude over the mother's or father's attentiveness to each other or new partners, particularly if the physical expressiveness is very apparent as may well happen with new relationships.

Again, if the situation does not seem to resolve itself and is causing a lot of distress, ask for help.

LYING

To some parents lying is a concern, to others it is not. Children who are afraid of their parents' reaction to what they say or do will naturally tell more lies. So a vicious circle is likely to be set up if the one thing that most upsets and angers the parents is their child telling lies. If a family gets into this kind of situation professional help will probably not aim solely to stop the child telling lies but to intervene with the family overall.

MASTURBATION

Masturbation used to be a major reason for admission to a mental institution in the Victorian era, then for referral to a child guidance unit in the 1930s. It is now rarely a great source of concern even though sometimes a bit of anxious public masturbation is not uncommon in five- to seven-year-olds. Sometimes, however, this can be a sign of and a source of worry for the child him or herself.

MISERY

'Miserableness' sounds like an irritating state – although obviously closely connected with unhappiness. If you yourself as a parent can't find out what it is about, and it seems to persist, then ask for help. Children often genuinely do not know or cannot say what is troubling them, and they may need the aid of someone outside the family.

NAIL-BITING

Nail-biting is another symptom that is no longer fashionable as grounds for referral to a child guidance unit. This is very sensible as research shows it is more common than not in children of about 10.

'NERVOUS' HEADACHES AND TUMMY-ACHES

Some children display signs of stress in bodily symptoms such as tummy-aches and headaches rather than mis-behaviour. The first port of call for help will probably, therefore, be your GP or school doctor. (See also Chapter 6.)

NIGHTMARES AND NIGHT TERRORS

If a child is suffering from nightmares, he or she may wake up, perhaps cry out in distress and recall something of a frightening dream. This sometimes has a repetitive theme, often of being chased or attacked by monsters or witches. This is particularly common at about the age of seven.

With 'night terrors' the child screams and may appear shaky and frightened, but is not clearly awake, does not speak of a dream and does not recall the event in the morning.

Such events may be normal or a reaction to unusual stress, and are usually grown out of. Sometimes it is necessary to exclude the possibility of epilepsy and if there are other persistent signs of emotional disturbance or distress as well, it is sensible to ask for help.

OBESITY

If your child is very overweight, this will probably lead to teasing at school and may cause future health problems. Very occasionally the obesity is due to physical causes and this may need checking out. If you have seen your GP and/or a paediatrician or school doctor then the school nurse or a dietitian may be the health professionals most likely to be able to help, advising and supporting your son or daughter towards a more healthy pattern of eating. Psychological treatments are rarely more successful than this in the long term, but attending a group such as Weight Watchers (see Useful Addresses on page 239) can be helpful.

OBSESSIONALITY

Many young children like the comfort of little rituals rigidly stuck to, such as 'Mummy kiss teddy and elephant and baby kangaroo and hippo goodnight'. A very few are distressed by any deviation from routine at any time of day and sometimes, if associated with other signs of speech or social delay, this is a characteristic of the child with autistic features. Older children sometimes have 'obsessional thoughts' which they cannot get rid of, and may behave in strange ways such as repeatedly washing their hands or having to check things over and over again. Such a situation can be differentiated from what is loosely called 'obsessional tidiness' by the distress caused if the ritual is not followed, and would certainly warrant calling in professional help.

OVERDOSE TAKING

Intentionally taking an excessive amount of some medication is not uncommon teenage behaviour. Usually, but not always, it is a girl and there is often a situation of some immediate social upset such as an argument with parents over a boyfriend, or stress such as exams. It may seem an angry gesture rather than one that is definitely suicidal, and sometimes engenders annoyance rather than sympathy from the family who may feel unjustly attacked. It is worthwhile, however, for parents to swallow their pride and go along with the help that is offered by the GP or hospital – usually referral to a social worker or the child psychiatry department. Sometimes therapy in a crisis like this can quickly achieve a great deal in helping families improve their capacity to sort their problems out more constructively, hence the expression 'a cry for help'.

SADNESS

Of course, sadness is a normal human emotion in situations of loss, of a relative, friend or even a pet, or feared loss such as if a parent is ill or long absent. Sometimes it takes people outside the family such as a teacher to notice or hear about a child's unhappiness. If you and your child can talk together about the reasons for the sadness, then probably all will be well. If you find this difficult, perhaps because of stresses you are under yourself, then additional help may be useful.

SCHOOL FAILURE

See Chapter 7.

SEEING GHOSTS

Perhaps because the experience of death is less common and much more concealed nowadays, you may not be aware of the very strong and strange emotions and altered perceptions that may arise from bereavement. This can include thinking that you can see and or hear the person who has died, particularly perhaps at night, and it can be very frightening to a child. Adults usually don't 'believe in ghosts', but think how commonly they are the subject of books, comics and television shows for children. Listening to and accepting the child's account and providing any necessary extra temporary comfort will help this phase to pass.

SEXY TALK OR BEHAVIOUR

These days open sexual scenes or discussions are common on television, and swearing is endemic in most play-grounds. At the same time society has become much more aware of the possibility of child sexual abuse.

If your child's school raises this as a source of concern, think through carefully how it might possibly have arisen and try to sort out with the teachers what approach would be best. When children's behaviour is embarrassing to talk about, like this, it is difficult for parents not to either over-react or under-react.

There may be some need for a school-based programme of health education which you could support the head teacher in asking for. If the school is so worried that they wish to notify social services, then it is still best to co-operate as much as possible, but also consult your own GP.

SHOP-LIFTING

Shop-lifting is a common minor delinquency, often committed by groups of young teenagers for the thrill of the risk as much as the material gain. The least sophisti-cated member of the group is, of course, the one most likely to be caught. If you are the unlucky parent, then your anger and the penalties of increased supervision (grounding) are likely to be as effective as anything. Don't waste your breath asking why – you won't get an answer.

SHYNESS

Shyness is a personality trait which can seem unusual to an outsider, but normal to a family where everybody is rather similar. 'Elective mutism' is an extreme version in which a child typically behaves and speaks quite normally at home but in outside situations, such as school, refuses to speak at all. This could be a sign of underlying worries but is particularly common at the stage of starting school, especially if another language is spoken at home, and usually passes off gradually. If it doesn't or you are especially worried, seek help.

SLEEP DISTURBANCE

It is perhaps the disturbance of the *parents'* sleep that is the main problem here. If your child will not go to bed or stay in his or her own bed, this can cause havoc in a family. When you have decided to tackle the problem, both parents will need to join forces for a systematic approach. Books can be helpful (e.g. Jo Douglas and Naomi Richman, *My Child Won't Sleep*) and often there is a local health visitor or clinical psychologist running a sleep clinic where you can find expert advice and support. Medication should not be necessary.

SMOKING

For health reasons it is important for parents and schools to try to prevent children even from experimenting with cigarette smoking as it is an extremely addictive habit. If you discover, nevertheless, that your child is smoking then a one-off health discussion with the GP or school doctor is well worth trying. Supervision and setting a good example are also worth the effort.

SOILING OR 'ENCOPRESIS'

Children are usually 'clean' in the sense of using the potty or toilet for defaecating by two-and-a-half, although expert self-wiping takes longer. Some children take a lot longer to develop this control and others seem to relapse.

It may be difficult to discover which came first, but a fear of the toilet and constipation are often associated. Battles between parent and child may then ensue, with the child seeming to refuse 'to go' on purpose then later 'pooing their pants'. Slightly older children sometimes hide their soiled underwear too. Go to your GP or local children's health clinic for help in the first instance, as simple measures can be effective and there are sometimes special clinics for soiling and enuresis. If the problem is very persistent and disturbing, then if physical factors have been excluded, more definite psychologically-oriented help should be sought.

STAMMERING

Stammering or stuttering are sometimes just hesitations evident when a child is developing language skills. If this becomes distressing for the child or you find you are beginning to react in an irritated and counter-productive way, then a speech therapist is the person to consult. They usually work at your local child health clinic or development centre. Ask your health visitor, clinic doctor or GP.

STEALING FROM HOME

Some parents regard taking food from the fridge without first asking as stealing while others do not mind children taking money from their purses, so family definitions are important. Is it secretive? What happens next? Is the child taking money to 'buy friends' at school for instance, or to finance an addiction? If you want things to change you will probably need to make clear the household rules, and try to learn from your child what pressures he or she is under in case there are things you can do to help. If such behaviour persists it may become very difficult for parents to tackle by themselves. Referral to a child guidance clinic would be appropriate.

SUICIDAL TALK OR BEHAVIOUR

Sometimes children as young as five or six may talk of killing themselves or wishing they were dead, and this can be very difficult to evaluate or understand. Obviously it is best to err on the side of caution and assume there is a serious issue behind the statement, unless you are certain it is just being lightly copied from television or neighbouring adult behaviour. Although children under the age of 13 rarely actually kill themselves, the point to consider is why they might feel so unhappy as to be thinking about it. Outside help is certainly warranted.

SWEARING

Another normal behaviour – in its right place. Extremely rarely, swearing can be compulsive and uncontrollable and may be accompanied by sudden compulsive movements. This is known as Gilles de La Tourette Syndrome and can usually be helped to some degree by psychiatric treatment.

TEMPER TANTRUMS

Temper tantrums are a particular feature of the two-year-old stage when the drive for independence is not matched by verbal development and competence. Often when the child learns other skills of getting his or her point of view across the tantrums diminish. But not always! If it is about a demand, give in quickly or not at all. Otherwise you are training your child to escalate the problem. If you have a temperamentally difficult and sensitive child this advice is far from easy to follow, but professional support can help.

TICS

A tic is an involuntary movement, often a twitch of the face muscles, and is most common in boys of about 10. It may be a sign of anxiety in the first place. Like other habits which are irritating to others, teasing and demands to stop it make matters worse. A rare and severe form occurs in Gilles de la Tourette Syndrome (see swearing above).

TRUANCY

Truancy or 'bunking off' is very common in the last years of secondary education, especially amongst children who are not successfully engaged in the course work for the GCSE exams. Take it very seriously and work with the school to overcome the problem (see also Chapter 7).

UNTIDINESS

'Not tidying his or her room' is not so much a symptom of a child's disturbance but of a battle between parent and child. If you are finding behaviour of this type particularly enraging and a cause of rows, then green hair and razor-slashed jeans will probably be the next things to keep you on the go. Think about what you are trying to achieve. Obedience? Helpfulness? Self-reliance? Or even getting the room tidy? This will make it easier to negotiate what to do next with your son or daughter. Consider how your relationships are always shifting – how you would approach the situation with a two-year-old – and with a 25-year-old!

WORRYING

If a child seems unaccountably and unusually withdrawn and worried, try to find out what it is about. Quiet, stubborn children often do not readily tell people what is on their minds, and then cannot easily communicate when under a severe stress. See if a teacher shares your view and has any clues as to what is happening. If a major problem develops, such as school refusal, or if you remain puzzled or concerned, then a child guidance unit will be able to help.

WRIST-CUTTING

It is usually girls rather than boys who cut their wrists, a situation which is sometimes described as a tendency to 'inwardly' rather than 'outwardly' directed aggression. Although the motivation is not usually actually suicidal, it reveals considerable inner pain which seems to be relieved in this way. There is already likely to be great family distress, conflict or breakdown, and wrist-cutting unfortunately tends to lead to admission to an institution of some kind, where it may get even worse. So, if this happens in your family get the best possible professional help as soon as possible.

2

PROFESSIONALS AND AGENCIES

One of the reasons it can be difficult to find help for the emotional problems of children is the variety of names quite similar services may go under, and the complicated titles of the professionals involved. The following is a guide to the most common terms.

ART THERAPIST

As the name implies, art therapists aim to help people through artistic expression such as painting or pottery. They are specially qualified and there are not many working with children within the NHS. Referral would probably be via a child psychiatry team.

BEHAVIOUR THERAPIST

This is a less common term. Usually psychologists, psychiatrists or nurses who have had special training use behaviour therapy as one of their techniques. A behaviour therapy approach in suitable cases, for instance, might be to encourage children to think about or face in reality situations which they are avoiding through anxiety.

CHILD GUIDANCE UNIT/CLINIC

Child guidance units or clinics may be found in premises owned and administered by either the National Health Service or the local authority, and typically have employees from both. A common pattern is for there to be child psychiatrists from the health authority, educational psychologists from the education service, and social workers from either education or social services. These professionals will vary as to how much they work together as a team or separately, but they can form effective links between the different services and get to know the local community well.

Referral policies vary: you may be able to walk in yourself or telephone for an appointment, or your child may have to be referred through your GP or the school.

CHILD PSYCHIATRY DEPARTMENT/CHILD AND FAMILY PSYCHIATRY DEPARTMENT

Child and family psychiatry departments are usually also multi-disciplinary clinics, but sited in a hospital. They are likely to have child psychiatrists and clinical psychologists, and sometimes also nurses and child psychotherapists. There may be hospital social workers from the local authority attached.

These departments may be more specialised than the community clinics and able to provide access to intensive day or in-patient treatment. There are usually good links with the paediatric services.

Referral is usually through the GP or paediatrician.

CHILD PSYCHIATRIST

A child psychiatrist is a medically qualified doctor who has undertaken further specialist training in general and child and adolescent psychiatry. The training posts in the NHS are at registrar and senior registrar grade; the consultant is the most senior. There may also be assistant specialists in child psychiatry.

CHILD PSYCHOLOGIST

A child psychologist is a graduate in psychology who has undertaken clinical training in general and child psychology before specialising. While in the past they mainly assessed a child's development, now they also offer a variety of therapeutic approaches.

In many places a GP can refer directly to a child psychologist. They may also be part of a child psychiatric team.

CHILD PSYCHOTHERAPIST

A child psychotherapist has undertaken special training to treat the problems of emotionally disturbed children. They are concerned with the child's inner thoughts and feelings and the unconscious mental processes of which the child is not even aware. Child psychotherapists are relatively few in number and are mainly based in London, working in NHS hospitals and clinics and also privately. Treatment usually requires a commitment of regular weekly attendance for the child for perhaps a year.

CLINICAL MEDICAL OFFICER (CMO)

A clinical medical officer is qualified in medicine and usually works in the community health service, taking sessions in schools, baby and toddler clinics and sometimes also family planning. Their expertise is, therefore, in the normal development of children. As school doctors, they often provide counselling for children and parents and usually know about resources to help with emotional difficulties.

CLINICAL PSYCHOLOGIST

A child psychologist is a specialist clinical psychologist. Sometimes the expression 'clinical' psychologist is used to differentiate between psychologists who have trained within the Health Service and educational psychologists (see below).

CLINICAL PSYCHOLOGY SERVICE

Some health authorities offer services for children from clinical psychologists as part of the main clinical psychology service. Referral is usually from the GP.

COMMUNITY PSYCHIATRIC NURSE

Community psychiatric nurses are a fairly recent development and there are only a few working in child psychiatry, though this is likely to increase. As the name implies community psychiatric nurses (or CPNs) are trained psychiatric nurses who have undergone further experience and training delivering treatment within the community rather than only in hospital.

COUNSELLOR

Anyone can advertise themselves as a counsellor, so you should try and find out the counsellor's qualifications and ask around for recommendations before approaching one.

EDUCATIONAL PSYCHOLOGIST

Educational psychologists have training, qualifications and experience in both teaching and psychology. They usually work within local authority education services as part of the School Psychological Service. Their roles differ in emphasis from place to place, but they usually offer advice to schools and sometimes also to parents and children about children with learning difficulties or emotional problems which affect school attainment. They have a major role in the Full Assessment procedure for special educational needs provision (see Chapter 7). Referral is usually through the school, though sometimes parents are allowed to make a direct approach.

EDUCATIONAL SOCIAL WORKER OR EDUCATIONAL WELFARE OFFICER

Education social workers (previously known as education welfare officers) work for education or social services. Their major responsibilities are school attendance, and liaising between school and home if it seems that home problems may be affecting a child. (See also Chapter 7.)

EDUCATIONAL THERAPIST

Educational therapists are usually teachers who have had further training and use their understanding of a child's anxieties to help them overcome their learning difficulties.

FAMILY CENTRE

Some child guidance units are called family centres, but this term is also used for social services' or voluntary agency provision for helping families with very severe difficulties in coping. Access is then usually via social services.

FAMILY THERAPIST

Family therapy is a technique widely used by different professionals in child psychiatry and child guidance. There are specific training courses and sometimes family therapists are employed to specialise in that technique only. Usually the whole family is required to attend, at least initially, and the focus is on the relationships and communication between all members of the family, not just the 'problem child'.

HEALTH VISITOR

Health visitors are trained nurses with a further qualification. They usually visit all mothers with new babies and provide advice at infant welfare centres and health centres. They often work closely with clinical medical officers and GPs. Increasingly, they may have links with the local child psychiatry and psychology services, and may offer sleep clinics, parent discussion groups and so forth. They can be a very useful source of support and information for the parent with young children.

HYPNOTHERAPIST

Hypnosis or hypnotherapy is sometimes requested by parents for their children and can be very helpful. Like other therapies, some professionals use variations of hypnotherapy techniques. To be certain that your child is receiving a professional approach, it is sensible to make sure that any therapist is either working in a reliable and well-known setting or is well qualified and recommended.

OCCUPATIONAL THERAPIST

Occupational therapists have a general professional qualification in occupational therapy. Some go on to specialise in work with children and provide vital help and support to sick children in hospital. Some may undertake further training, such as in counselling, and become part of multidisciplinary child psychiatric teams.

PAEDIATRICIAN

A paediatrician is medically qualified and has further experience and qualifications in the assessment and treatment of children. Most paediatricians work in hospitals with out-patients and in-patients. Community paediatricians have responsibility, as the name implies, for the organisation of children's medical services in the community, such as immunisation programmes, developmental assessment, baby and toddler clinics and advice to education and social services. Referral is through the GP or the health clinic or school doctor.

PLAY THERAPIST

Play therapy may be undertaken by different mental health professionals. Occasionally in children's services there are dedicated play therapists who are likely to have had training based on psychodynamic theory. Play is a useful way of understanding the inner world of the child, and can offer an opportunity for a disturbed child to work through his or her problems.

PSYCHIATRIC SOCIAL WORKER

Traditionally, the psychiatric social worker worked as part of the child guidance team taking a special role in understanding the family and community aspects of problems and working particularly with the parents. They are qualified social workers, often with further training in psychotherapy for children, families or adults.

Unfortunately, pressures on social services to provide rapid responses to emergency work especially for children at risk has meant a decrease in the availability of a longer-term therapeutic approach.

PSYCHIATRIST

A psychiatrist is medically qualified and has gone on to gain further training and qualification in problems of the mind.

PSYCHOANALYST

A psychoanalyst may or may not be medically qualified, but has had extensive training in the treatment of psychological problems based on the theories of Freud, Jung or Klein. Some specialise in the problems and treatment of children. The treatment is usually long term and may have to be paid for privately.

PSYCHOTHERAPIST

'Psychotherapist' is a slightly vague term, literally meaning someone who treats problems of the mind. Make sure if you are approaching a psychotherapist that you are referred by someone who knows they are reliable and that the psychotherapist has a suitable professional qualification, and belongs to a reputable organisation.

REMEDIAL TEACHER

The term 'remedial teacher' is now a little old-fashioned, but a teacher was often part of the team at a child guidance unit, offering one-to-one or group-work help to children with learning difficulties (usually with reading) based on emotional or concentration difficulties. Such teaching is also sometimes available in schools.

SCHOOL NURSE

School nurses are qualified nurses who undertake a specialist role in schools. They do a lot more than eye-tests and first aid and are often approached by parents and children for advice about a variety of worries.

SOCIAL WORKER

A social worker usually works for the local authority social services or for a voluntary agency. The term covers people with an extremely wide variety of training, experience and skill, but usually the agencies they work for have extensive knowledge of the local problems facing families and will try to help. They may refer you on to other more specialist agencies such as child guidance or may be able to help directly themselves.

3

HOW TO FIND HELP AND WHAT TO EXPECT

HOW DO YOU GET YOUR CHILD REFERRED?

If you are worried about your child's behaviour or adjustment, you can raise this with your GP, health visitor or clinic or school doctor. Their advice may be the next thing to try, or they may suggest that your child is seen at a child guidance clinic or its local equivalent.

If so, ask about the clinic or service you will be going to. For instance, does your GP have a leaflet about it? What are the alternatives? Sometimes it may be best for your child to be seen at a clinic which has special links with education, or it may be best to go to a clinic which works closely with the hospital paediatric services. Does the GP know what kinds of approaches are likely to be offered? If you already have firm preferences about this, let the GP know.

Having agreed with you where the child should go for treatment, the doctor will probably write a referral letter to describe the problems. In some places the local policy is for the parent to contact the clinic directly, in which case the doctor will give you the address and telephone number.

It may be that the school has noticed that there is a problem. In this case the school, after communicating with you and gaining your agreement, will write direct to the local child guidance clinic itself.

WHAT HAPPENS NEXT?

Usually, within the clinic, the referral letter is looked at by what is called a multi-disciplinary team – that is a group made up from people like a child psychiatrist, psychologist, social worker, psychotherapist and perhaps a community psychiatric nurse. The composition of the team varies from place to place. Members decide which combination should be assigned to see the child and how urgent it is.

Some clinics will send you an appointment letter straight off, others may write and ask for more information or ask you to complete a form. Some clinics write or telephone to check that you are still interested in receiving an appointment, or ask you to send back an appointment confirmation slip. This is because clinic staff set a large amount of time aside to see your child, and quite a lot of people change their minds about coming – whether because the problem has improved or because of cold feet!

The appointment letter should give you some idea of who and what type of professional person you will be seeing, and it may indicate how long the first appointment is likely to last – usually about one-and-a-half to two hours.

You may well be asked if the entire family living at home can attend. If that is difficult to arrange then you should ring up the department or clinic to explain. It may be a matter of timing: the father, for instance, can't come until after 4 pm, or a sister has an exam on that day. The clinic will often try to be flexible about the time in order to see as many members of the family as possible because it has been found that doing it this way saves time for everybody in the long run.

You may think that the school is going to be very upset or worried about any child having to take time off to go to the child guidance clinic. But schools know the general policy of these clinics and they are almost always helpful and supportive in arranging for any child with a problem to have the necessary time off to attend the clinic, along with any brothers and sisters in the family.

Sometimes, if your child has a complex problem in which other agencies have been involved, the clinic may ask for permission to contact them before the appointment. For instance, a school report may be needed or the child's medical history from another hospital. The clinic may also get in touch with the referrer for further information if it thinks it necessary.

HOW SHOULD YOU PREPARE?

Children sometimes arrive at the clinic very anxious and it emerges that they have thought they were going to be punished or left there because they have been so bad. After all, a child is almost bound to realise that it is something about them having been naughty or upset that is the reason for coming. Perhaps to prevent unnecessary anxiety you could be open about that – reminding them of the particular incident or perhaps the visit to the doctor that had made you decide to seek help for the worries affecting the family. Say that everyone has come along to try to help and mention what you are all going to do immediately afterwards – like go home for lunch, or to the shops. The details you should go into depend, of course, on the age of the child.

Because the interview may be fairly long, or there may be a short wait first, it is sensible to bring along essentials for very young children such as toys, snacks or drinks and nappies.

WHAT HAPPENS AT THE CLINIC?

Your appointment is always individually booked, unlike an out-patient appointment where there can be 50 other people booked at the same time. It is therefore important to be on time as you are normally seen very close to your appointment time.

On arrival, usually a receptionist will take any further details necessary, such as checking your names and dates of birth and address. Sometimes at this point a family is asked to fill out a form for some further information. The waiting area is usually fairly pleasant, with magazines for the adults and toys and comics for the children.

WHO DO YOU SEE AND WHO SEES YOU?

Usually, the person – or people – who will be interviewing you come to the waiting area, introduce themselves and accompany the whole family or the individuals they are going to see to an office or interview room. The person conducting the interview will also tell you who is listening in and watching this interview. This may sound rather 'Big Brother-ish' but sometimes the interview room is set up with a one-way screen which looks like a mirror and allows what is happening in the lighted interview room to be visible, through the screen, from the adjacent darkened room. (If a light was put on in the darkened room, those in the interview room could see the watcher.)

The professional will not only explain exactly who is on the other side of the screen – like a colleague or a trainee – but also what the purpose is of their observation. When a professional is assessing a whole family, it is quite difficult for them to do it on their own because of the subtle inter-actions that take place between family members. It can be difficult for them to keep their eye on five people at once and so it's helpful to have the observations of an otherwise uninvolved colleague as well. Sometimes two professionals share the interviewing and again both will explain who they are.

You may see a video camera in the room, which may or may not be on, and this should also be explained. Some-times it is helpful for the children to know what is going on and they may be allowed to have a quick look at whoever is next door so they can see how the system works.

You should be asked for your agreement to the inter-view being watched or recorded and you may want a fuller explanation of why it is helpful. For instance, students learning about child psychiatry may be watching; or if a trainee is conducting the interview it may be necessary for a supervisor to be watching; or a trainee may need to watch a more experienced colleague. Sometimes the inter-viewer is wearing an ear-bug, through which he or she is receiving specific instructions or advice from someone on the other side of the screen, acting as supervisor.

WHAT HAPPENS IN AN INDIVIDUAL INTERVIEW?

Sometimes the parent or parents are interviewed separ-ately from the child, either by different people at the same time or by the same person in turn. Parents are likely to be asked what their concerns were about the child that brought them to the clinic, and to give as much detail as possible about the problem and what they have already tried. They may also be asked for information about the child's early experiences and development and about all the members of the family. They are also likely to be asked if there have been any major recent stresses for the child or family, and perhaps to tell the interviewer about their own experiences of childhood.

Parents often feel quite anxious – thinking that they will be blamed or that the clinic will want to know about their sex lives. But the questions and listening at length to what parents have to say are often very helpful as the cause of the problem or why it has not been easily overcome may not be clear beforehand.

What may be happening to your child meanwhile? Depending on the age of the child, their interview may be rather like that for an adult – with questions and encouragement to talk about their point of view – or they may be encouraged to communicate through play or drawing. There are always toys available such as small dolls and dolls houses, cars, bricks, puppets and so forth. Some of the toys, such as puzzles, are designed to help assess a child's developmental level, others to help them to feel relaxed and perhaps begin to reveal what is on their minds.

If you or your child has been interviewed separately the full details of what each of you has said will not be disclosed to other members of the family without permission.

WHAT HAPPENS IN A FAMILY INTERVIEW?

The way that family interviews are conducted varies

widely. Sometimes questions are addressed mainly to the parents, but usually other members of the family – especially the child principally concerned – are asked for their view or account of what happened. Some interviewers like to obtain a full detailed history at this stage, others encourage the family to communicate and interact with each other as this often brings out the nature of the difficulty.

For instance, if you are discussing something like an argument between you and your partner and the children start a noisy diversion so that you can't even hear what each other is saying, the therapist may get a clue as to why such bad behaviour starts.

At the first interview, after about 45 minutes and whether or not a full history has been gained, the interviewer may take a short break to confer with colleagues on the other side of the screen. At this point the mirror is covered and the video turned off. You may be wondering what is going on! The professionals will be discussing what they see as the mainsprings of the problem and what more needs to be known or asked about – either from someone else involved or from the family, as the problem may be complex. They will also be thinking about what kind of advice to offer.

After the break, the psychiatrist, or whoever is conducting the interview, may need to ask one or two more clarifying questions. Then they will tell you what their first impressions are of the nature of the problem. They will also discuss with you what kind of further action you can all mutually agree on.

WHAT HAPPENS AT THE END OF THE FIRST ASSESSMENT?

At the end of the assessment the professionals discuss the next step with the parents. It may be that further assessment or investigation is necessary. Another appointment may be made for you to come to the clinic again so that a longer history can be taken. A psychologist's assessment of the child's intellectual attainment may be carried out separately.

The professionals will discuss their first impressions with you. Sometimes, with some sorts of problems, this is like a medical diagnosis, but may be more of a general appraisal of the varieties of stress experienced by the child and family and how everyone has responded.

HOW IS THE TREATMENT AGREED?

Sometimes further family discussions are offered which are likely to be helpful, but may be fairly open-ended as to their subject matter (goals of treatment often shift). Sometimes the focus for help needed is clear and particular arrangements offered, or 'goals' may be agreed with the parents and children, and perhaps tasks or 'homework' set.

HOW LONG WILL TREATMENT LAST?

Be sure to ask about this if it is not made clear. Sometimes one interview may be enough or all that you want, especially if understanding and perhaps advice or reassurance is what you are looking for. Additional advice to the school is often also helpful.

A common arrangement is the offer of about six family interviews over the course of a few months with the opportunity of a review after that. Sometimes weekly or fortnightly individual interviews for the child and/or parent are offered.

Clinics vary as to how flexible they are about the times and lengths of treatment, but there is usually some chance of negotiating these.

WHAT ABOUT PRIVATE TREATMENT?

Sometimes you may hear about private treatment from friends, or it may be recommended by your GP or by the clinic you first go to. Clinics, for instance, often have to spread their resources thinly among the many cases in need and if it seems that it would be best for you or your child to receive long-term individual psychotherapy or counselling they may recommend going privately and will know who to suggest.

Individual professionals and organisations, especially in London, offer a variety of treatments and usually make clear which type they can offer before the consultation is arranged. The advantage of this option is that you may have less time to wait and you should have a good idea of what type of treatment to expect. You may also feel that you are not being 'made' to go, as it is more under your own control. Make sure that you get as much information as possible about who you are going to see or about the organisation. Not all GPs know about these resources, but it is sensible to get a recommendation from somewhere, not just answer a newspaper advertisement. Questions you should ask include: what is the training and background of the therapist? What professional organisation are they attached to?

WHAT ABOUT CONFIDENTIALITY?

Often in the kinds of interviews discussed above, many little discussed, sometimes painful or embarrassing feelings or events are revealed. Interviewers do not tell even another member of the family what has been revealed to them in confidence, but an interview in which everybody is present gets around this problem. Every professional and the secretarial staff understand that what they are told must be confidential and the professionals will discuss with the parents what information will be helpful to share, for instance with the school. Your GP is usually advised of the result of the assessment and of the proposed course of treatment.

An exception is made to the rule of confidentiality if there seems to be a risk to the child. Then the professionals have a duty to share their concerns – usually with the social service department. Even so it is good practice to keep the parents fully involved and informed.

4

COMMON CAUSES
OF PROBLEMS

If a child's behaviour changes it is very often due to outside influences. It may be, for instance, because of family stress before or after parents divorce; or it may be a reaction to stress at school, such as bullying; or it may be a response to bereavement.

The following are typical case histories of children who have been brought by a parent for help at a child guidance or child and family psychiatry clinic. They show the different kinds of problem that affect and distress a child, and how families may react to reasonably common, though upsetting, circumstances especially when these are combined with several other stresses.

FAMILY MOVES

Robert, aged seven and an only child, was brought to the child guidance clinic by his parents at the suggestion of his headmaster.

His father had been in the army since before Robert's birth in Germany. The family stayed in Germany until Robert was three and then moved to England. The family moved to Hong Kong when he was nearly five and Robert went to school there. He behaved so aggressively at this school that he was very nearly expelled.

After two years the family moved back again to London where at school he appeared cheerful but, according to his headmaster, was very disruptive and also very easily distracted. His class teachers reported that he was attention-seeking and behaved provocatively. He was rather a loner and was wary with new children, though later would attempt to dominate them. He was very easily upset by criticism at the new school.

His father was expected to be in the army for another two years, and also saw himself as a loner and prone to fight. He himself had been taunted at school. Robert's mother accepted army life, with its constant moves and her husband's absences. Neither she nor her husband could account for their son's difficulties in school. His activeness and his wariness were acceptable behaviour at home.

When Robert was asked questions about the way he behaved at school he was at first reluctant to answer. A rather sad-looking boy, he was asked if he knew what a worry was and in reply he described how he remembered thinking his parents had left him on a beach – an idea which considerably surprised his parents. He also described how 'horrible' his previous head teacher had been and how he used to lose his temper and fight when he was called names by classmates – he had obviously found this upsetting.

When he was given some toy soldiers to play with and was asked to choose one to represent his father, Robert set him up in a well-protected position and used a plane to vanquish the enemy entirely.

Comment

Army families, as well as the soldiers, may be expected to 'be brave' and not make a fuss when subjected to stresses such as frequent, involuntary removal from their known environment, and often having their father away perhaps in an unknown location and subject to uncertain dangers which he may not even be allowed to speak about afterwards. This little boy obviously had considerable anxieties that he had not previously been able to discuss with his parents and unfortunately this was being compounded by his difficulties in settling in at a new school.

◆

Sean, aged six, was referred to the child guidance clinic by a paediatrician at a London teaching hospital because he was wetting and soiling and was often excessively shy in company, refusing to speak to strange adults.

He had been to several different nurseries and nursery schools and was very shy and unhappy there. He had been at his present school for about six months, becoming gradually more confident. Sean's parents were from Ireland. His mother was an anxious woman who very much identified with Sean because she herself used not to speak to people because of a stammer. She was still shy and socially isolated and had become depressed and irritable because since marrying seven years previously she had left her own country and family to live in constantly poor accommodation, while her husband had difficulty in getting steady employment. The family – the parents, Sean, two younger brothers and a younger sister of 18 months, were living in a three-bedroom flat with serious damp. Even that was an improvement on their previous lodgings.

The family background was one of stress in almost all areas: housing, financial and marital. Sean himself was a temperamentally anxious child who reacted to the prolonged family and social stress with shyness, wetting and soiling. As his mother's depression lifted he himself started to improve.

Comment

This is a story of one family's experience of immigration and its strains. Sean's symptoms of shyness, wetting and soiling revealed an insecurity made worse by the repeated changes of home and education which he had to undergo. As his total family situation began to change for the better, Sean's signs of disturbance also began to lessen. His mother very much identified Sean with herself and one might speculate that he had been expressing her distress as well as his own.

◆

FAMILY CONFLICT

Jason, aged six, was referred by his GP because he had been behaving badly at home and at school and had started to wet his bed again. He was the elder of two children and there was no contact with his own father. His mother's current boyfriend, and father of the younger child, was frequently violent to the mother and had also threatened Jason. The mother had taken an overdose on at least two occasions, but although offered psychiatric help had not taken this up.

At the clinic, Jason's mother seemed quite depressed and agreed that the priority was not so much to 'treat' Jason's understandable disturbance as for herself to get the support she needed to sort out her family situation.

Comment

Children suffer from domestic conflict and violence even if
they themselves are not the direct victims. If they seem to
have the most public symptoms – perhaps of insecurity or
aggressiveness – it can, sometimes at least, serve the useful
purpose of bringing help to the overall situation.

——————— ◆ ———————

Jean, aged 12, was referred because of reluctance to go
to school, and poor progress and lack of friends when
she was there. She came to the clinic with her mother
only. Her parents were separated and her older brother
aged 15 had refused to come. It turned out that the
brother terrorised his mother and sister, actually hitting
them if they did not instantly obey him in every respect.
The father had refused to intervene and the mother did
not protect her daughter.

Comment

'Parent-bullying' like this does occur, but is a source of
such shame that it is rarely acknowledged. This particular
example again illustrates that the referred member of the
family may not be the one who is most disturbed nor in
most need of help.

Little change can be expected in a situation like this
unless the adults are willing to take steps to regain appropriate authority. Separated parents may find it hard to
collaborate effectively, and a deserted mother may find it
hard not to try to bring back her husband by having family
crises, so it is worthwhile seeking help even though the
way to progress will not be easy.

——————— ◆ ———————

PARENTAL SEPARATION AND DIVORCE

Emma, seven-years-old and an only child, was referred for child psychiatric help by her GP.

Her father had walked out, without any warning, on Christmas Day two years previously and had gone to live with another woman. Since then Emma's personality had changed. She had become much quieter, was often withdrawn and her mother found it difficult to communicate with her. She was particularly upset when, as often happened, she was let down by her father arriving late for visits, or not appearing at all.

Her mother had been devastated by the marriage break-up, but said she 'had to be strong for Emma'. Although she had tried to keep her anger hidden, she admitted to hating her ex-husband for what he had done to her daughter. She clearly saw Emma's problems as psychological, but blamed all these entirely on her ex-husband.

When being assessed at the child and family psychi atry department Emma paused a long time before answering questions, although she spoke fluently enough on subjects of her own choosing. She drew an idyllic picture of a little girl standing among flowers with the sun shining and said this was not her but a younger child from school. When asked to draw an opposite picture, she produced a drawing of a little girl standing in the rain. The girl was crying and holding an umbrella which only partially covered her. Emma would not explain anything about either picture.

Comment

Emma's reaction to the separation of her parents was clearly the reason for her withdrawn behaviour and

disturbed emotions. Nearly all children feel very sad, ofte
angry and even guilty if their parents separate. They find
especially difficult to accept that either parent is 'all bad
and find it hard to have to take sides even when one of th
parents seems to be behaving very irresponsibly. Emm
did seem to be finding it hard to communicate her feeling
about this and perhaps her mother's well-intentioned but
misleading 'bright front' was contributing to this.

◆

Adam, aged 14, was referred to the child guidanc
clinic by an educational psychologist. His mother an
father had separated seven years previously and h
father had remarried while his mother shared a hous
with her boyfriend. The atmosphere was tense as sh
didn't allow the boyfriend any authority over the tw
boys (Adam had an older brother) although he wishe
to be protected from their noise.

Adam was very much indulged by his mother. H
had poor concentration and was easily bored. Althoug
quiet and polite to other adults, he had violent row
with his mother if he was challenged.

In order to avoid rows his mother stopped insistin
that he went to school, and over the last two term
Adam had only been to school for one or two days
week, although his attendance had improved somewh
when he went to a special small teaching unit in th
grounds of his school. Adam's mother had not forcib
taken him to school, used any sanctions or even show
any anger at his behaviour. She felt it was up to her so
whether or not he went to school. His father, who live
nearby and whom Adam could visit whenever he chos
agreed.

Adam's father, who came to the clinic with his e

wife and the children, retreated from questions about his responsibility for his son. Adam said very little when they were all at the clinic, but he seemed very pleased at his father's rare expressions of interest or anger.

Comment

Parents often need help in exerting their authority over their children jointly and consistently. This becomes even more complicated when the parents are separated and there are new partners. It appears kind to a possibly unhappy child not to insist on their doing things that they may find inconvenient or even stressful, but this can be a very short-sighted option. It seems here that both parents were trying to avoid provoking any overt expression of Adam's distress and anger, perhaps in order not to be cast in the role of the 'bad parent'. However, this may have been felt by Adam not as kindness, but as a lack of concern and an ignoring of his painful feelings about the situation.

◆

Katy, aged six and an only child, was referred to the clinic because she was pulling her hair out, not doing what she was told and generally behaving defiantly. Her mother had left Katy's father two years before to go to her parents because he had been violent since she married him and also had a drink problem.

Since the couple had split up there had been disputes about the time and amount of access the father had. Katy had not seen her father for several months. The last time she had done so he had shown her his new baby. The mother had a new partner, whom she was hoping to marry, who was mainly around at weekends.

When Katy was asked about possibly being unhappy at home she said that because they hadn't got a dad, her mum was too busy to read to her. Everyone else had a dad and a baby. To her mother's obvious distress, Katy said that she thought her father didn't care about her and gave his money to his girlfriend's children instead.

Katy then drew a crying lady whom she 'made happier' by drawing in teeth. Sometimes, she said, she was angry with her father and would like to punch him in the eye or teeth. She drew a bottle of alcohol and said 'It makes people drunk and then they fight'.

Comment

Katy had been reduced to pulling her hair out. The fact that her mother and father had both found new partners was no comfort to her – indeed quite the reverse – especially when she became displaced by her father's new baby. She also communicated more than her parents realised that she would; she did remember the drinking and the violence and she was angry as well as unhappy.

◆

ACCESS PROBLEMS

Georgina was 10 when her mother brought her to the child guidance clinic.

After a deteriorating marriage, Georgina's mother had left her husband two years previously. The mother had custody and Georgina and her younger brother were allowed to stay with their father every other weekend and at Christmas.

In the few months before she was seen at the clinic,

Georgina had shown signs of becoming increasingly upset when she returned from weekend visits to her father. She would cry, have migraines, did not want to go to school and was so reluctant to go to sleep that she had to be settled to sleep in her mother's bed. The mother and father quarrelled about Georgina's state as the father did not agree that Georgina was upset.

At the clinic Georgina drew pictures and later told the story. She drew a picture of a tower in a wood. It is Christmas, there is a star in the sky and it is snowing. There are ghosts in the tower, stuck there because of the snow. A little girl comes with her dog and goes into the tower. She believes that ghosts can be friendly. When she goes home she gets lost in the snow and the ghosts rescue her. Georgina admitted that she felt panicky when she came home from her father and would cry out for her mother.

Comment

This child is evidently being disturbed by the access visits to her father's home. If this is the tower in the story, clearly the little girl has some positive feelings towards it as well as anxieties. However, it is the custodial parent, in this case the mother, who has to make up her mind how best to act for the sake of the child. This mother decided that it would be best for access visits to cease, and Georgina did become more settled. Nevertheless, there is evidence that for many children it is helpful for their better emotional health later to keep up contact with the non-custodial parent.

Daniel, aged nine, was sent to the child guidance clinic by his school's clinical medical officer.

His father had left his mother two years before for another woman and the father visited the children – there were five beside Daniel – only irregularly.

After his parents had separated, Daniel, who had been very close to his father, began to suffer from night terrors. About four times a week he would sleep-walk with his eyes open, looking confused and frightened and saying 'Oh God'. His mother would comfort him out of this and allow him into her bed, and afterwards he did not recall anything. When by himself Daniel was always fantasising, pretending to be Batman or another super hero.

His mother complained of her ex-husband's irregular visits, which caused tension in the family, and was afraid he might even kidnap Daniel.

Comment

Daniel was showing a common childhood symptom of distress – night fears and separation anxiety. Why this child was the most obviously troubled of the family is not quite clear, but it is interesting to note both that he was very close to father and also taken by his mother into her bed. Possibly he was always seen as special in some way, and, as in a previous case, the child with whom a parent particularly identified.

This can make it very difficult to work out sometimes how serious a child's difficulties are in their own right and how much they are serving as a form of communication for a parent. In this case the mother wanted the child's symptoms to be used as a justification for preventing her ex-husband visiting the home, but it seems more likely that this was about her own wishes than Daniel's.

———— ◆ ————

SEXUAL MOLESTATION

Christine, aged eight, was referred to the clinic by the voluntary association Victim Support. She had been sexually assaulted two months before by a man known to and trusted by the family.

Christine had initially cried a lot and had then become very defiant; she had become reluctant to attend school because the assault was known about and she was teased, especially by older boys. She was angry about this, saying that she would like to kick the boys concerned. Her mother, depressed since the incident but unable to talk about it to her husband or to Christine, told her that she should forgive the boys. The father had tried to beat up the molester and the assault had made the whole family feel disturbed.

Comment

While tears and withdrawal after a severe trauma such as an assault may be accepted, sometimes parents find anger hard to understand, especially if directed towards themselves. Often old emotional wounds of the parents are opened up and for this reason they find it especially difficult to be available to help their child sufficiently, or perhaps to communicate effectively with each other. In this case it was evident that the marriage was being put under a great strain.

◆

Lorna, aged nine, came to the clinic with her mother at the suggestion of a social worker.

Lorna's mother had noticed that she had become very withdrawn in the presence of her mother's

boyfriend and had lost weight. Because the mother ha
other suspicions she eventually went to the police
Their talk with Lorna revealed that she had bee
sexually interfered with on several occasions by th
mother's boyfriend.

The mother told the boyfriend to leave the hous
and Lorna was reassured by her mother's ange
although she couldn't describe her own feelings clearl
Lorna remained rather more quiet and anxious than sh
had been previously.

Comment

Lorna's mother had intervened to protect her daughter i
a most responsible and efficient way, but while the girl'
disturbance remitted rapidly the mother remained ver
depressed, self-blaming and angry with her ex-boyfrien
She had to decide whether to go ahead with allowing he
daughter to be a witness for the prosecution when th
chances of successful conviction were unknown and th
court experience was likely itself to be traumatic fo
Lorna.

Such lingering uncertainties before a trial takes plac
are unfortunately only too common and mean that eve
an initially short-term experience of an event such a
assault can continue to have an on-going impact for year

◆

Hayley, aged six, was taken to see the child psychiatri
at the hospital clinic after two incidents of a sexua
nature. In the first she was 'felt up and kissed' by a ma
in a supermarket while her mother had left he
momentarily unattended. Two weeks later a man o
the estate where she lived, known to be an alcoholi

and drug abuser, exposed himself to her. On both occasions the mother had informed the police and court cases were pending.

Since these two happenings, Hayley insisted on sleeping in her mother's bed, demanded her mother's constant attention and had become very 'clingy'.

When seen by the psychiatrist, Hayley held on to her mother. She had been kidnapped from her mother by her father when she was only a month old (the parents had separated by then). Both Hayley and her mother were eager to talk about their problems and seemed rather frightened and insecure.

Comment

It was not clear that Hayley herself would have reacted as badly to these events – unpleasant as they were – without her mother's reaction. However, from the history of the early 'kidnapping' one can see that the mother understandably had particular anxiety for this child and was doing her best to protect her. Sometimes reactions such as this also indicate experiences from the parent's own childhood from which they are now trying to protect their own child.

◆

BEREAVEMENT

Mark, aged 11, was brought to the child guidance clinic by his mother after he had played truant with older boys for a week before half-term and had then refused to go back to school afterwards. Mark would not say why he disliked school.

His father had died two years previously and Mark

had refused to go to school after this had happened. When asked if he knew of anyone who had died recently, Mark said that a man living in the same block of flats had done so, and in fact his uncle, to whom he was very close, had just killed himself. He admitted to the psychiatrist that he was worrying about his mother, frightened she might get knocked over or fall down and be killed.

Comment

Although this case may sound extreme, it is striking how often parents fail to realise that a bereavement in the family may be strongly affecting a child as well as themselves, no matter how secretive or reassuring they try to be. As often happens with cases of school refusal, Mark is not so much afraid of school as anxiously preoccupied with what might be happening to his mother. This is often called separation anxiety and can be as strong a feeling on the parent's part as on the child's.

◆

Victoria, aged seven, was brought into the child guidance clinic by her mother, who was worried about the tantrums she had been throwing for the previous six months. The school had also complained that she had bitten another child and was often aggressive.

In the months leading up to Victoria's behaviour changing for the worse, it turned out that her grandfather had died suddenly from cancer and a long-standing nanny had left. There had been several other changes, including the fact that her mother had taken on more responsibilities at work.

At the clinic the mother revealed how very distressed

she had been by the death of her father and how she was still coming to terms with this. Victoria became quite agitated and told her mother that she shouldn't be upset as she should know that she would see her father again in heaven.

Comment

Children, like adults, often have to face change and loss. It is when everything seems to happen at once that it becomes difficult to cope. Open sadness seems to be difficult for this family judging by the little girl's reaction to her mother, so perhaps that is why she herself, not really understanding what had been going on, was driven to biting and aggression.

◆

David, aged 15, was referred to the child guidance clinic by an education welfare officer. He came to the clinic with his father, his mother having died six months previously after many years of severe illness.

David had been playing truant, lying about where he had been or was going, and had been involved in delinquent behaviour. He had been picked up twice by the police for shooting air-rifles and for carrying out criminal damage in a primary school.

His behaviour had worsened considerably after his mother's death and at the clinic he seemed depressed and frozen, answering almost every direct question with 'I don't know'. His father admitted that the two of them had not really discussed his mother's death.

Comment

Sometimes the death of a close member of the family, even if long expected, can make people so upset that they cannot communicate with each other and therefore fail to complete the tasks of mourning in the usual way. This may be the case particularly if there are mixed feelings about the loss – for instance of guilt or even relief. An outside observer might not immediately recognise David's misbehaviour as an expression of his concealed grief – yet looking at the time sequence this seems the most likely explanation.

◆

Stephen, aged 12, was referred to the child guidance clinic by Victim Support. He had been mugged two months previously and forced to give up his money at knife-point.

This had brought about a resurgence of the symptoms that Stephen had suffered when his father had died two years before. These included wetting the bed three or four times a week, difficulties in getting to sleep, over-sensitivity about school, having rows with his mother and blaming her for his father's death and thinking about this death a lot.

The reason Stephen blamed his mother for his father's death was because his parents had had a row the night before his father died and they had not slept with each other. Finding him dead the next morning, the child believed it was his mother's fault and his relationship with her, though close, remained tense.

Comment

Frequently, quite severe symptoms may be triggered off by a fairly minor stress, while the main 'causal stress' occurred some years before. Stephen's feelings of renewed insecurity appear very clearly here and his mother, now a single parent, has found she needs help and reassurance in coping with her distressed son.

◆

SECRETS IN THE FAMILY

Wendy, aged 14 and an only child, was sent to the child guidance clinic by her GP. For the past two years she had withdrawn from her parents' company at home, going off to her room, reading and listening to the radio.

More recently, she had become increasingly moody, leading to two incidents in the previous months of her attempting to cut her wrists. The first time she said it was because her jewellery had been stolen; the second time because of a boyfriend. The parents said that Wendy did not want to talk about her reasons for cutting her wrists and was always very secretive.

Wendy's mother was a moody woman and, it eventually emerged, an alcoholic. She had involved her daughter in covering up her drinking and her debts to hide the situation from her husband.

Comment

Wendy was part of a family which superficially looked as if it was functioning well, but in reality its members were not communicating and had considerable hidden pain.

Wendy wanted to keep her parents together and protect each of them, but her own distress 'leaked out' through the wrist-cutting.

———————— ◆ ————————

Richard, aged 13 and one of five children, was brought to the child guidance clinic by his mother, who had separated from her husband some four years before.

The problem was that Richard had taken to playing truant from his school more and more. He would go off alone and, it was thought, to his father's flat. He was also spending a lot of time at a friend's house without telling his mother where he was. When questioned about his activities he would shout and swear and lock himself in the bathroom. He had also stolen small sums of money from members of the family, although he did not seem to spend it. His mother had sometimes threatened to send him to live with his father but had never carried out this threat.

Richard said that he worried a great deal about both his father and his mother and felt he had to go and see how his father was. His mother thought he was very like his father, who also lied and stole, but Richard argued that his father was nice and he could not see why his parents had separated. He had not been told that his father had sexually interfered with his two older sisters.

Comment

In this case, although understandably, the child had not been told the true reason for the divorce by his mother – who did not tell the therapist at first either. Richard too, had his own secrets – where did he really go? What exactly did he spend the stolen money on? His parents were finding it very difficult to get together to secure Richard's safety, let alone his school attendance. Sometimes even professionals cannot find out exactly what is going on, but try to build some framework of trust and acceptance so that the family can at least start to think about serious and worrying issues like sexual abuse. Often years later, a family member or the child when grown up may think of going themselves to a therapist, and may then describe how they couldn't talk about the issue previously.

◆

Tom, aged six, was referred to the child guidance clinic by his GP. His parents had separated the previous year because, according to his mother, she had been unable to tolerate his father's habit of bringing friends into the house and not being responsible for them.

On being asked, Tom said his mother had not told him why his parents had parted. After the separation Tom's father visited the home every two weeks. When he did he spent most of his time just watching television. Tom seemed very upset after his father's access visits, becoming devious, destructive and telling lies. The tension between him and his mother was so bad at times that she had to leave the room and this was getting worse.

At school, Tom, who was a bright boy, showed increasing unhappiness, aggression and a tendency to lie.

His mother eventually admitted that she had been an alcoholic and still attended AA meetings. Tom's father also had a long-standing drink problem and went on binges. Tom, who was liable not to answer when asked questions, did comment that he thought being drunk was 'crazy'.

Comment

Families in which alcohol dependency is a problem often try to cover up and present a more perfect picture of family life even to themselves. In this case the child knew that both parents had alcohol problems, but had probably not been previously allowed to say so – especially to an outsider. Creating the possibility of open communication turned out to be more important than the apparent question of whether access should be stopped as useless or too painful.

◆

PHYSICAL ILLNESS IN THE FAMILY

Philip, aged seven, was referred to the hospital clinic by an education social worker. He had been behaving destructively – gouging the wall with a knife, for instance, and cutting up clothes. He claimed to hate his mother, behaved badly towards his brother and sisters when his parents weren't looking and was generally disobedient and hyperactive.

His problems started when he was about two-and-a-half and his mother was in hospital for three months because of a difficult pregnancy. When mother and baby returned Philip was obviously jealous and hit his sister with a broom. His sister turned out to have a serious liver disease requiring repeated hospital admissions, so this naturally meant that she continued to need a great deal of their mother's attention.

Comment

The usual pangs of jealousy over a new brother or sister were heightened for Philip because the baby seemed to have made his mother stay away from home for a long time. When, in addition, the baby needed lots more attention because of prolonged severe illness Philip seems to have had to go to extremes to convey his feelings, but unfortunately this only made matters worse for him.

◆

Ruth, aged four, was referred to the child guidance clinic by her GP.

She had always been a sensitive child but was now throwing tantrums and refusing to settle at bedtime. If allowed downstairs, she would eventually sneak into her parents' bed. Her behaviour particularly annoyed her mother as she would put on her mother's shoes, use her make-up and draw on the walls.

Ruth wet the bed when upset and had bad nightmares about witches who boiled children in pots. Her problems had become much worse since her mother had had a severe bout of colitis the previous year.

Comment

Ruth's signs of disturbance do seem particularly related to her mother. With a severe physical illness, which in this case was not especially visible, a parent can seem suddenly to withdraw from a child for no reason. Children also often pick up the fears and feelings of others, perhaps about cancer, without being able to put this into words.

◆

Sharon, aged 10, was sent to the child guidance clinic by her doctor, who could find no physical reason for her symptoms.

Sharon was having 'turns' in which she felt hot, anxious and that the walls were looking at her. She wouldn't let people touch her; she would go pale and blotchy and cry. Her parents became very distressed at these symptoms and were worried that she might be having fits.

Sharon was the youngest of a large family of children and was rather spoiled as a result. The preceding year her mother had been ill with high blood pressure and although at the clinic Sharon denied worrying about her mother, an older sister, who was also attending, reminded her that she had been.

Comment

Sharon's turns sounded very severe and worrying, but in fact improved rapidly with some discussion of the family anxieties and advice to her parents on how to handle the symptoms. Worrying about Sharon's 'turns' seemed to have provided an alternative for the family to worrying about the mother's high blood pressure, which might in fact have had a more sinister significance.

———————— ◆ ————————

Lucy, aged seven, was referred to the child guidance clinic by her GP.

A quiet child, she had been found stealing her mother's jewellery which she had taken to school and had given away. On discovering this her parents had kept her in and the head-teacher made her give up her favourite dolls for a week, but the same thing had happened again.

The previous year, Lucy's four-year-old brother had developed diabetes and had to have daily injections. Lucy started to tell fantastic stories at school, even claiming both at school and at Brownies that she herself was diabetic and had to be injected with a needle. At the clinic Lucy was outspoken and defiant, boasting of how she lied to her parents and teachers, read when she shouldn't, had given her brother sweets and so on. She challenged her parents and later said of her brother: 'I hate him'.

Comment

Lucy has not only been displaced by a new baby but in addition he is given lots of attention for being ill. Lucy tries various methods to re-establish herself – including claiming to have the same illness as her brother, taking things from her mother and being generally naughty and angry. Fortunately, although this behaviour was highly irritating, Lucy's parents were able to see the connections and be sufficiently sympathetic to Lucy to ask for help.

◆

MENTAL ILLNESS IN THE FAMILY

Martin, aged nine, was referred to the child guidance unit by his school's educational psychologist.

He was being difficult with the teachers and not getting on well with his work despite remedial help. At home he worried about his mother, and night-time anxieties and bad dreams often led him to join his mother in her bed.

Martin's father's relationship with his mother had lasted three years, then he was imprisoned for drug offences. Since then he had been mentally ill, needing hospital admission at times. He came round to visit Martin, but his threatening and unpredictable behaviour was alarming.

In the interview at the child guidance unit Martin was mainly cheerful, but readily recounted his recurring nightmare that his mother was being chased and caught by a monster. His mother was holding a responsible job, and had no family nearby.

Comment

Severe mental illness of a parent can have a number of different effects on children. There can be the worry of a direct genetic link – will the boy turn out like his father? There is the loss of a competent parent, putting responsibility for all aspects of family maintenance and child-rearing onto the other parent. And there can be the stresses of dealing day-to-day with the unpredictable, sometimes violent behaviour of a mentally ill family member. Martin and his mother did not have much external support and their family situation was one of considerable strain. The source of Martin's nightmares is plain and it is likely that anxiety was also affecting his ability to concentrate and learn at school.

◆

Pauline was 15, the youngest of four children, and came to the clinic with her mother.

She had been referred by the educational welfare service because she had not attended school at all for several months. She described how even thinking of school made her ill, how she had quarrelled with all her friends and was afraid of teasing. Her parents had separated five years previously, but kept in touch over major decisions, although the father was said to disapprove of work and school for philosophical reasons.

The second child, Simon aged 26 and still living at home, had had two schizophrenic breakdowns and was under continued treatment. Discussion of his illness was stressful for both mother and daughter, but the symptoms included general aggressiveness and a loss of ability to work and care for himself adequately.

Comment

Pauline wanted to continue to get some education, and the education welfare officer was able to sort out an acceptable, less challenging solution for her. Her brother's illness had not only contributed to her own anxiety, but had also impaired the capacity of her parents to cope with any extra problems.

5

IS MY CHILD...?

This chapter gives details of some major patterns of childhood psychological disturbance that most people will have heard of, and may be wondering if their own child falls into one of the categories. It is worth remembering that there are fashions in diagnoses. In the nineteenth century neurasthenia (nerve weakness) was the thing to have, and now myalgic encephalomyelitis (ME) has become an increasingly used label. Doctors use diagnoses to help work out how to prevent diseases, what treatments are commonly most effective and what the likely prognosis or outcome will be. A recurring pattern of symptoms is sometimes called a syndrome.

IS MY CHILD ANOREXIC OR BULIMIC?

Anorexia nervosa

This is a condition that affects mainly girls. Have you become aware that your daughter is:

- Becoming obsessed with slimming magazines, with the calorie content of food, or with trying out different diets for a longer time than normal?
- Constantly on the bathroom scales and angry or

highly anxious at the suggestion that they be thrown out?

- Starting to miss meals because of various excuses, such as the fact that she has just eaten, is eating later with friends, doesn't like what is on offer, is not feeling hungry, has just eaten, or is on a particular diet that needs private preparation?
- Always eating a very small amount or spending meal-times pushing food around her plate and hiding it under other food like lettuce leaves?
- Tending to wear bulky sweaters or floppy, concealing garments so that her actual size is not apparent?
- Refusing to go to the doctor for a check-up or admit that anything is wrong?
- Suddenly taking a great deal of exercise, like walking to school, jogging, running up escalators?
- Missing periods or has stopped menstruating alto-gether?

If you have noticed examples of the above behaviour, it is very possible that your child has developed anorexia nervosa. Anorexia comes from the Greek, meaning loss of appetite, but in fact anorexics fiercely resist eating because they either want to lose weight or are overwhelmingly fearful of putting it on, and not because they are not hungry. Nor is their aversion to the food itself, but to the effect it will have on their body shape.

Anorexia usually starts after the onset of menstruation, but in a small number of girls it appears to be triggered off before then by the advancing signs of puberty and so can occur in nine and 10-year-olds. Studies have shown that about one in 100 school girls are anorexic; fewer boys are anorexic, possibly because they are less concerned with their shape.

Anorexics are often very bright, middle-class girls who are apparently high-achievers but may secretly lack self-esteem. Triggers may include an anxiety-provoking sexual experience, teasing about their body and worries about their parents' marriage. They may find that although they originally wanted to slim to conform to modern ideas of beauty, they then enjoy the successful feelings of control over their own bodies that results.

But although they start with this feeling of control, they in turn find they are controlled by their need to lose weight. Even if their weight drops to six or even five stones they regard themselves as being fat when they are, in fact, emaciated. This severe loss of weight naturally has other effects on the body: lack of sugar can cause dizzy spells; blood pressure and pulse rate drop; respiration is slow; poor eating causes constipation.

Referral to a specialist psychiatric service is essential as young people can and do die from anorexia. Sometimes admission to a hospital is necessary to ensure proper nutrition, but sometimes the condition can be managed successfully by out-patient treatment. Currently there is good evidence to show that, for the young anorexic especially, family therapy treatment can be very successful. It is not uncommon, however, for there to be some residual problems and a need for further therapy may arise later.

Bulimia

Bulimia is often referred to as 'second stage anorexia' but it is generally known as bingeing. What happens is that anorexics who have kept a fierce control over the intake of their food find that their resolve suddenly cracks and they turn voraciously to eating food – particularly carbohydrates – which they have been totally avoiding.

To counteract this sudden bingeing, the anorexic/bulimic immediately makes herself vomit up all the food she has eaten or purges herself with laxatives. She then goes on an even more severe diet to make up for what she regards as an appalling lapse of control. And so the vicious circle of starving and stuffing goes on. Bulimics also realise that bingeing at least allows them to eat some food rather than constant self-starvation.

Bulimics are very frightened people as they feel – quite rightly – that their eating has got completely out of control. They compulsively binge and then starve – and then go on to gorge on cakes and a dozen or so bars of chocolate. There is no pleasure in this kind of eating: it is just a physical cramming in of as much food as their body will take. Sometimes the food is obtained by obsessive shop-lifting, as part of the need to keep their behaviour secret.

Bulimia is a more difficult condition for parents and others to recognise, and is less life-threatening than pure anorexia nervosa. However, it is a significant distortion of adjustment and also needs expert help.

Case histories

Katie was 14 when she happened to overhear a giggling remark about her weight when she was at a disco. She wasn't in any way obese, but she was plump. She also lacked confidence socially, even though she was very bright academically. Her parents had high hopes for her and she was under pressure to do well with school work.

She felt she wasn't being asked to dance because she was too fat and wasn't attractive enough. She went on a diet for a week, lost a few pounds, but found she still wasn't particularly popular as a dancing partner. This depressed her. At meal-times she pushed food around but ate practically nothing, and then started disappearing at meal-times, saying she was eating with a friend. She started getting up at 6 am to do an hour running before school.

She was convinced that if only she could lose enoug weight she would be more sought after. She also fe that as she saw the arrow on the scale start to fal entirely through her own efforts, that she was in contro for once and not just a puppet obeying her parent wishes.

Her parents, though constantly telling her to 'eat u and stop being silly' were hardly aware that her weigh had plummeted to near five stones as she wore larg baggy sweaters. When they did realise it they did nc know how to cope. Katie collapsed several times an was admitted to hospital where they insisted she at and supervised her during meals. Katie put on weigh was discharged from hospital and promptly lost weigh again. She was readmitted and only when she was see by the hospital psychologist, who explored her ir securities and helped her change her attitudes, did sh begin to recover.

◆

June, aged 16, is an example of how an anorexic ca conceal her condition. She made very plausible excuse as to why she was always missing meals, like: 'I hav just eaten', 'I'm eating later with friends', 'I'm nc feeling hungry now.'

When she did eat it was always a very small amoun or she would push food around her plate and hide under lettuce leaves. If her parents commented, sh snapped at them, so they tended to leave her alone. Sh also made a point of wearing bulky sweaters or floppy concealing garments so her actual size was neve apparent.

When her mother happened to catch sight of her coming out of the bathroom one day and insisted she went immediately to the doctor, she first of all refused. When she finally went her weight was not as bad as the mother feared. It turned out, much later, that she had deliberately weighed herself down by putting a lead weight in her jeans.

June also obsessively over-exercised, weight-lifting and jogging constantly until she was too weak to do so.

———————— ◆ ————————

Frances, aged 16, had not been through an obvious phase of anorexia nervosa, but had unsuccessfully dieted and then regained excessive weight (in her own opinion) and was secretly very preoccupied with food and her weight. She had become an expert at making herself sick quietly and effectively after a large meal, and had learned to use laxatives.

Sometimes she would gorge herself; one lunchtime she ate five chocolate bars, a cheese and pickle roll, a sausage roll, a doughnut, a fruit yoghurt, a piece of cheesecake, two packets of crisps, two soft drinks and a bag of chips. Before this she ate some carrots so that she would be certain, when she finally vomited up these carrots, that she had got rid of absolutely everything she had binged on.

None of her friends or her parents guessed what was happening. It was her dentist who alerted her parents when he noticed that the acid from her constant vomiting was rotting her teeth.

What parents can do

The real problem facing parents is that the anorexic does not consider anything is wrong with her. Above all, she does not want anyone to treat her as she overwhelmingly wants to go on controlling her intake of food, to keep it to a minimum amount. She is likely to argue furiously with her parents about every mouthful, be quite irrational about her appearance and strongly resist going to a doctor. Parents are going to have to be quite tough about this and avoid getting into bargaining mode, with the anorexic constantly failing to keep her side of the bargain – i.e. to eat.

When the young anorexic is seen by a psychiatric service, it is very likely that the whole family, especially both parents, will be asked to attend. Even though 'whole family' discussions can be painful, they are necessary in this instance. Instructions given to the whole family also need to be followed; try not to get into a battle with the therapists, or with each other, as your child will by now have become an expert at playing one person off against another. You may also have to face issues about your marriage which you hoped were concealed from your children but turn out not to have been.

Often the battle is fought kilogram by kilogram, particularly as the weight which heralds the onset of menstruation is approached. Keep going.

Probably the best advice is to ask for specialist help early, and to make every effort to overcome the problem, rather than hoping it will go away or leaving treatment when there is a partial success only. Then be aware that there may be a relapse or the development of bulimia. Parents whose children have been anorexic and have apparently recovered should watch to see if their child disappears to the loo after a meal or is hiding food in their room. If so, specialist help is needed again.

Useful organisations

There are various self-help organisations (which both parents and child can attend) that can be helpful. All the organisations which help anorexics will also help bulimics.

Eating Disorders Association
(previously Anorexic Aid)
  The Priory Centre
  11 Priory Road
  High Wycombe
  Buckinghamshire HP13 6SL
  Tel: 0494 521431

Helps and advises sufferers of anorexia and bulimia nervosa, families and friends through voluntary self-help groups.

Eating Disorders Association
  Sackville Place
  44–48 Magdalen Street
  Norwich NR3 1JU
  Tel: 0603 621414
  Youth helpline: 0603 765050

Offers help, support and information.

IS MY CHILD AUTISTIC?

Autism

Autism is a condition in which a child seems to be withdrawn into himself – hence the name. It was given wide publicity through the film *Rain Man* in which the adult autistic, played by Dustin Hoffman, shows some of the characteristic anxieties and odd social behaviour. Autism is rare and there is some disagreement between professionals as to which children should have this diagnostic label. For instance, mentally handicapped children commonly have autistic features too, and some children who have rather odd personalities with shyness and obsessionality are sometimes regarded as being within the 'autistic spectrum'.

A child with autism may seem to develop fairly normally until about the age of one-and-a-half to two years, when speech, instead of developing rapidly into short but meaningful phrases, remains at a few single words only. Then 'echolalic speech' may appear in which the child repeats what is said to him instead of forming new sentences of his or her own – 'Does Mikey want a biscuit?' instead of 'I want a biscuit'.

Normal two-year-olds like to be sociable – to chat, play and squabble with other children, and to enjoy friendly approaches from adults. But the autistic two-year-old seems not to want to share human contact but to avoid it, and will often look away instead of smiling in response to a friendly adult glance (known as gaze avoidance). Close observation may show that the child's play is more often repetitious than imaginative and even minor deviations from routine cause anxiety leading to temper tantrums. Some children behave in a repetitive self-stimulating way such as flicking their fingers in front of their eyes.

From two years onwards development varies. Most autistic children need special education and intensive help to get them as involved as possible with normal life, and sometimes considerable psychological help is also necessary to help them overcome their socially handicapped behaviour.

About half later develop epilepsy which contributes to the probability that autism is a physically based condition, rather than due to poor early mothering as once thought.

The outcome in adult life is related to how much language is eventually acquired. Many autistic people used to end up in institutions and sadly some still do. Nevertheless a lot more is now known about how to help such people live as normal a life as possible.

Case histories

Esther, aged three, was referred to the child psychiatrist for delayed speech and difficult behaviour. She turned out to use very few words, preferred to sit in her buggy and pulled at her parents to get what she wanted. Her main form of play was piling things up and she largely ignored the other children at her nursery school. Her parents had to let her do what she wanted – such as keeping on her coat – or she would scream. At this early stage the diagnosis could not be certain, but became more and more clear as the months passed with little progress despite considerable help from the school, the psychologist and the speech therapist.

◆

Louis' failure to speak was noticed by child guidance staff who were treating the family because of concerns about an older child. By three he did not speak at all despite normal hearing, and normal development in physical skills. At home he was very destructive, active and difficult to control. He was always poking things into the electric sockets and screamed if he did not get what he wanted. He needed a great deal of attention and was admitted to a day child psychiatric unit for under-fives and from there to a special school for autistic children attached to a ordinary primary school. Specialist staff attached there included a child psychiatrist, an educational psychologist and a social worker and there was also a high teacher-pupil ratio.

At the age of 11 Louis progressed to a nearby boarding school for autistic children.

———————— ◆ ————————

Arthur seemed to have had a reasonably early normal development, but was simply never interested in other children. He was precociously able in mathematics and obtained a scholarship to a private school. Even at his interview, however, he was thought to be rather odd as he tended not to look anyone in the eye and paused a long time before answering questions. Unfortunately his perfectionism made him unable to complete home work demands on time and eventually the school insisted that he leave. At the age of 13 he began to see a child psychotherapist regularly and it became clear that though very intelligent, he did not at all understand concepts of human emotions and relationships and was often very puzzled by what was going on around him.

At 16, his unusual personality characteristics continued, together with a capacity to exasperate his parents and teachers. He is considering whether to take a college course in a science, but may again find it difficult to comply with the normal institutional demands.

What parents can do

It is always a dilemma to know when and what to 'label' a child. Autism used to be sought as a label by parents who thought it might be a marker of hidden genius in what could otherwise turn out to be a mentally-handicapped child. Sadly autism is a very real and disabling condition which will have implications for the whole of a child's life and that of his or her family. Louis, above, was severely autistic, and Esther less so. Arthur did not gather that particular label, but nonetheless needed special educational provision and therapy and had an unusual personality of what some would call 'autistic type'.

Parents do need to be aware of any unusual development in their child's language and social behaviour and make sure that an assessment is carried out and followed up. In some districts health and education authorities collaborate at a developmental assessment centre which has the advantage of all the necessary expertise being gathered under one roof. If you are worried about the possibility of autism, do say so, for if this diagnosis is being considered it is helpful if the parents are fully informed and involved. Indeed, you are very likely to be asked to help in treatment programmes and often help is available for even some of the most difficult behaviour problems.

Under these circumstances parents often want to make sure they have exhausted every possible alternative diagnosis and treatment. Talk your ideas over with your GP or paediatrician. Sometimes a second opinion can be helpful. But beware spending too much time and energy on apparent miracle cures. Remember other people in the family must also be considered, as well as the unfortunate autistic child. Joining a group of parents can be especially helpful for mutual support, sharing tips about the system and keeping abreast of the latest knowledge about autism.

It is very likely that your child will need special education, and important that it is provided by those with special knowledge of the condition. While you are negotiating this, pay particular attention to what happens at the next stage. For instance, is there a choice of boarding or day education? What are the mechanisms for smoothing the transition to adult life? Remember that under the 1991 Children Act your child may be entitled to social services such as relief admissions or funding for special equipment. Your child's development centre or special school may have a social worker attached, or there may be a special team for disabled children – so do ask.

Useful organisations
National Autistic Society
276 Willesden Lane
London NW2 5RB
Tel: 081 451 1114
Provides information and education.

Scottish Society for Autistic Children
24d Barony Street
Edinburgh EH1 3JT
Tel: 031 557 0474

Provides help and guidance for parents of autistic children.

IS MY CHILD DELINQUENT?

Delinquency

Delinquency usually means the involvement by young people in anti-social and illegal activities. It is a general term, not a psychiatric diagnosis.

Delinquent behaviour might therefore include such things as shop-lifting, graffiti-writing, destruction of property, theft, joy-riding, setting fires, drug-taking and so forth. Anti-social, even illegal behaviour, is very common in teenagers, though much less frequently found out or brought to the attention of parents or police. Boys and young men in particular, if they start to 'hang out' together on the streets as a group or gang, may urge each other on to steal, destroy property, or fight another group.

There is nothing very mysterious about this. Any large group of similar people are likely to behave worse *en masse* than if they were on their own; think of MPs, or any company outing. However, even initially harmless situations can get out of hand, and vulnerable teenagers can find themselves in great trouble. If the first few incidents are not well handled then such teenagers may become more and more defiant towards their family and society.

The isolated delinquent, who acts alone rather than with a group, is at particular risk of a poor outcome.

Case histories

Dick had been out at a party with a group of friends. As they returned home late at night they decided it might be fun to climb over a fence and see if they could get into the sports club's swimming pool. A neighbour, aroused by the noise, called the police who took the boys off to the police station, searched and questioned them and found that two of the boys had marijuana on them.

Dick's parents were called and took him home. While his mother was inclined to ignore the whole affair, his step-father pointed out that this was just a culmination of events, during which Dick had become increasingly rude and argumentative at home and had got into trouble at school for silly behaviour and poor work. As the exam period was coming up, Dick's step-father insisted that Dick was taken to the GP, who referred him to the child guidance unit.

◆

Shelley was already attending the child guidance unit when she began to shop-lift and increasingly play truant. Her mother had only been 16 when she was born and was shortly afterwards put in prison for two years. During this period Shelley was cared for at her paternal grandmother's home.

When her mother came out of prison Shelley had a

period of unsettled care between several relatives and when she first came to the attention of the clinic, aged 10, her father and mother were fighting for her custody. Unfortunately, even when this was settled Shelley tended to run between the two when in trouble. Her worsening behaviour in her teens seemed to be related to the birth to her mother of premature twins.

A large family meeting was arranged at the clinic, the outcome of which was that Shelley returned to the care of her grandmother once again. A more settled period followed, but when Shelley was last heard from, at the age of 18, she had also been in prison and had a young baby.

◆

Vincent, 14, had been shop-lifting, playing truant and disappearing from home without saying where he was going. He was brought to the clinic by his mother, but not regularly as she kept hoping when things were going slightly better that no further help was needed.

As Vincent was very reluctant to speak, and the step-father refused to attend, it was very difficult either to understand the situation or to intervene effectively. Next the police found Vincent by himself at a railway station and his mother insisted he was taken into care. There he settled for a while, but never really revealed what had been going on. However, he established quite a good relationship with his 'key-worker', started to go regularly to a small educational unit and was able to return home successfully after six months.

What parents can do

Delinquency is not a single type of behaviour, nor has it a

single cause, so there are no simple answers as to what to do. First, how can you reduce the likelihood of delinquency in the first place? If your son or daughter is mixing with a group of youngsters that you know or suspect are capable of getting into trouble then do not just let it drift. Make clear your own values about drug-taking, damage to property and so on.

When both of you are in a good mood, discuss with your son or daughter what they want to achieve in later life and how they hope to do it. Ask if they have any particular worries, for instance about school, that you can do anything about. Make clear the household rules for your children – like coming in before midnight and always letting you know where they are. Become more flexible as they show their reliability and trustworthiness and increase freedom with age.

Try not to let one child in the family become the scapegoat – the one always to blame. If this seems to have happened then the child is unlikely to confide in you; but another family adult, such as an aunt or uncle, may be able to help.

But suppose you, like Dick's parents, get that call from the police station to say your son or daughter is being held there for some misdemeanour. A number of contradictory emotions often take hold, for instance:

- She is completely innocent, it must be the fault of her friends.
- The police have over-reacted.
- I warned her this might happen, why didn't she listen?
- She's been asking for trouble recently and deserves all she gets.
- This will kill her father (mother/grandmother, etc.) when he finds out.
- Will this be in the press? What will the neighbours/family say?

- It's all my fault for being a working mother/being divorced/having been too hard/too soft, etc.
- It's all her father's (mother's) fault for having left/been too hard/too soft, etc.

Share your chaotic thoughts and feelings with others, especially your partner and any other involved parents. The crisis is likely to pull all the members of the family in to help and may be useful to sort out failures of communication and renegotiate rules with your teenager. Try to remember that severe punishment, though tempting, is counter-productive and that one day you may all be able to look back on the incident and laugh.

If, on reflection, it seems that the incident might be a 'tip of the iceberg' issue – that is, though in itself minor, it draws attention to major underlying conflicts or unhappiness within the family – then ask for help through the child's school or your GP.

Useful organisations

National Association of Young People's Counselling and Advisory Services
Magazine Business Centre
11 Newarke Street
Leicester LE1 6SS
Tel: 0533 558763
Co-ordinates services for young people aged between 16–25.

National Children's Home Careline
85 Highbury Park
London N5 1UD
Careline (London): 081 514 1177
Careline (Birmingham): 021 456 4560
Careline (Leeds): 0532 456456

Careline (Preston): 0772 824006
Careline (Maidstone): 0622 756677
Careline (Taunton): 0823 277133
A phone-in service for people with family problems.

Young People's Counselling Service
 Tavistock Centre
 120 Belsize Lane
 London NW3 5BA
 Tel: 071 453 7111, extension 337

Youth Clubs UK
 Keswick House
 30 Peacock Lane
 Leicester LE1 5NY
 Tel: 0533 629514

Helps young people develop their physical and mental capacities.

IS MY CHILD DRUG DEPENDENT?

Drug dependency

One of a parent's greatest fears these days is that their child might become involved in taking drugs and that this might lead to 'dropping out', alienation from the family and society, a criminal existence, illness (possibly AIDS) and an early death. Parents are also aware that these risks are not confined to poor inner city areas, and that in most schools at least 'someone knows somebody' who can obtain or is using drugs of some kind.

Recent surveys have shown that many teenagers experiment with 'drugs' and consciousness-altering substances of many kinds – such as glue. What are they trying to do? They may be simply trying to imitate their friends and stay part of the group, or they may be trying to lead by appearing 'big' in doing something they know is disapproved of and possibly risky. However, the substances chosen are not accidental but can provide some sort of 'buzz' and excitement and a relief from everyday worries.

Serious problems begin to arise if the youngster turns to drugs solely as a relief from and a false solution to his or her life problems such as studying for exams, finding a job or making emotional relationships outside the family. As parental disapproval mounts, the teenager may leave home and find illegal or anti-social ways of affording to buy the drug. This is likely to include dealing and may clearly lead to brushes with the law.

After some years, often after repeated attempts to free themselves from their now unwanted habits, some drug-dependent young people do manage to limit their dependency or even give it up. Others may not manage to do this before irreparably damaging their health or their ability to get and keep a job.

Case histories

Jeannette was unhappy at home after her mother remarried and appeared to lose interest in her. Although she had been doing well at school she began to go around with a group of girls who were mainly interested in clothes, pop-music, parties and boys.

Jeannette met a boy who was several years older who admired her intelligence. He began to take her to discos outside the area, where drinking and limited drug-taking were common-place. The more trouble she got into with her parents for staying out late, dressing only in black, wearing extreme make-up and so on, the more Jeannette became convinced that only her new friends could understand her.

She left home and joined a squat at 16, and was soon

introduced to taking drugs intravenously. Occasionally she would return home, and try to 'get off drugs' but to her parents' despair this never lasted. At the age of 21, Jeannette found that she was pregnant and that social workers were considering taking the child away from her.

———————◆———————

Paul had been brought up by his mother only from the age of four and had one younger brother. Somehow it had always been Paul who was the focus of trouble in the family and he had also not got on well at school. From the age of 13 he preferred to be out with friends at a youth club, in a games arcade or just loafing about.

His mother rarely knew where he was in the evenings and Paul would give fairly evasive responses to questions, generally implying that his mother had no business to ask.

One day, when cleaning Paul's bedroom, his mother discovered what she knew to be marijuana as she had seen it used by friends herself when younger. She wondered whether to take it to the police but in the end decided to confront Paul with it – threatening to throw him out of the house if she ever found him using it again.

Paul told her that all his friends used it, that it was perfectly harmless and that anyway he was old enough to do what he liked. Of course he was not using hard drugs and had no intention of doing so. He pointed out that his mother smoked cigarettes and sometimes drank and that in his view it was just the same. An uneasy truce then ensued. Paul left school, and had a few short-term jobs. He left home to live with a girlfriend at the age of 18.

———————— ◆ ————————

Jeremy, at 16, was discovered by his boarding school to be part of a group that were experimenting with smoking dope (marijuana), and taking 'uppers and downers' – pills such as amphetamines and barbiturates. Two suspected ring-leaders were expelled immediately; Jeremy was asked to leave after taking his exams. Jeremy's father worked in the diplomatic service abroad, which was why the family had chosen boarding school to provide some stability for Jeremy in England.

Both parents flew back to Britain immediately and had angry but illuminating exchanges with both their son and his head teacher. It was eventually arranged that Jeremy would transfer to another boarding school to continue his education and that the family would consult a child psychiatrist in the holidays.

What parents can do

It can be a considerable dilemma for you as parents to decide how to react appropriately to your children taking drugs. Sometimes it just seems like the last straw in a deteriorating family relationship; sometimes it emerges as the explanation for withdrawal, pallor and loss of money from the house; sometimes the discovery comes out of the blue.

As with other types of misbehaviour, excessive threats and punitive restrictions may simply increase the teenager's dissatisfaction with their family and drive them away emotionally if not physically. On the other hand, it is very difficult for you to ignore such a worrying situation.

Do take the situation seriously and consider all the implications with your partner, family or friends. Is this an opportunity to repair family difficulties or personal unhappiness that have gone unresolved for a long time? Do you, the parents, try to overcome stress by drinking and smoking? Ask the school and your GP for advice as they may have come across very similar instances and know the best local source of further information or help.

The child guidance unit may not see many cases of this kind, but may well be able to help about general family difficulties, or know where to refer you. Beware of an immediate referral to an adult drug dependency service, as contact with older and more hardened users could simply make matters worse. Try your local town hall, health education department or social services for other suggestions, or one of the agencies named below.

Useful organisations

Adfam National
   1st Floor, Chapel House
   18 Malton Place
   London EC1N 8ND
   Tel: 071 405 3923
National telephone helpline for the families and friends of drug users.

Families Anonymous
   Room 8, 650 Holloway Road
   London N19 3NU
   Tel: 071 281 8889
Provides support groups for families and friends of those with drug or alcohol problems, or with an eating disorder.

Release (Legal, Emergency and Drugs Service)
   169 Commercial Street
   London E1 6BW
   Tel: 071 377 5905
Provides a 24-hour telephone advice and information service for drug-related problems.

Re-Solv: The Society For the Prevention of Solvent and Volatile Substance Abuse
    30A High Street
    Stone
    Staffordshire ST15 8AW
    Tel: 0785 817885
Provides information.

Turning Point
    Bedford Hall
    Bedford Road
    London W13
    Tel: 081 567 1215
Telephone counselling and practical help for those with drug, alcohol and mental health problems.

IS MY CHILD DYSLEXIC?

Dyslexia

Dyslexia can be defined as an unexpected difficulty in learning to read or spell; that is to say a child seems in other ways bright and developing normally, has reasonable concentration and general adjustment and has been exposed to good teaching.

There is evidence that this condition is associated with mild dysfunction of the left side of the brain and can sometimes run in families. Boys are about four times more likely to suffer from dyslexia than girls. The problem may persist in some degree even into adulthood.

Dyslexia was once called 'word blindness' and some education authorities currently refer to it as 'specific learning difficulties'. It covers a number of such difficulties, including: reversing figures and letters (15 for 51, was for saw); bizarre spelling; difficulty in recognising shapes; trouble in reading and in copying; confusing left and right; clumsiness; poor concentration span for reading and writing; bad memory; inability to remember multiplication tables; slowness at school work; lack of a sense of time.

Case histories

Jake was referred to the child guidance unit at the age of nine because of cheekiness and poor concentration in school. His parents, both of whom were graduates, came with him. They were more concerned that Jake seemed to be making little academic progress at his primary school and wondered whether he might be dyslexic. His uncle had had difficulties in learning to read as a child, so they felt this problem might run in the family.

Jake had been born prematurely and so there had been a lot of worry about him as a baby, although his later development had been normal. He had had an operation to lower one of his testicles at the age of five and because of this had missed some of the start of school. A baby sister was born at about the same time.

Psychological testing indicated that Jake was of above average intelligence, but his reading was just below the average for his age, his concentration was poor and so was his pencil control.

A variety of possible factors therefore seemed to have contributed to his difficulties. He was offered specialist one-to-one remedial help at the clinic for two terms, and benefited considerably.

◆

Ronnie's difficulties, especially with spelling, were noticed by both his parents and his school when he was seven. His parents gave him extra help with reading and spelling, but it became obvious that his younger sister was gaining on him and Ronnie was beginning to become self-conscious and reluctant to try. The educational psychologist at the school was asked to make an assessment and did think that Ronnie had specific difficulties. She recommended strategies for the school and parents to try, including using a computer, and also made available in school some extra teaching help for Ronnie.

◆

Ruth was referred to the clinic just after transfer to secondary school at 11. She had been known to the educational psychologist for some time because of her poor progress in reading. Her development had been normal and there seemed to be no specific deficits in the skills necessary for reading. She thus did not fit a pattern of dyslexia as a specific difficulty – yet still could not read.

Ruth's parents were separated, but she stayed with her father every weekend. She had an older sister of 15 who was mentally handicapped and went to a special school. In many ways, Ruth's skills had by now overtaken her older sister's and the most likely explanation for her reading failure seemed to be that she was attempting to maintain some degree of relative immaturity – and in terms of getting lots of attention for this, she was certainly being successful.

What parents can do

The signs of dyslexia such as letter reversals are normal and temporary phases for many children. However, even at the risk of being thought a fussy parent, it is worthwhile paying close attention to the progress your child is making in reading and spelling and giving lots of support at home without being critical. If you become concerned, discuss this with your child's teacher and head teacher. If there is a real problem they will have observed it too and you may be able to work on extra help together.

You can ask if there is more specialist help available – either a teacher or an educational psychologist – and it may even be worthwhile getting extra resources through the special education procedure. (See also Chapter 7.)

Sometimes parents are not satisfied with what is provided by the school – where resources can be quite limited. It is possible to get advice and help from organisations such as the British Dyslexia Association or a private educational psychologist. In most areas the Health Service's child psychiatry and clinical psychology services will be able to assess the nature of the difficulties, but are unlikely to be able to offer much long-term help of a primarily educational nature.

One-to-one specialist teaching can help most children with reading difficulties, whether or not there are the specific signs of dyslexia, but sometimes this label can be an advantage in getting an education authority to fund the provision and perhaps later in making any special arrangement for formal examinations.

Useful organisations

British Dyslexia Association
    98 London Road
    Reading
    Berkshire RG1 5AU
    Tel: 0734 668271
The overall national charity for dyslexia. It offers information and counselling for dyslexic children, their parents and teachers and a referral service.

Defining Dyslexia
    132 High Street
    Ruislip
    Middlesex
    Tel: 081 950 1033/868 6810
Provides a full, free support system to parents and children unable to cope with stresses caused by learning difficulties.

The Dyslexia Institute
    133 Gresham Road
    Staines
    Middlesex
    Tel: 0784 463935
Has a national network of centres and outposts which offer assessments, tuition, teacher training and support.

IS MY CHILD HYPERACTIVE?

Hyperactivity

The label of 'hyperactivity' has become much more common in recent years and is at least a way for parents to express and share their concerns when they have to deal with an unremittingly demanding and active young child (usually a boy). But is it a disease? Does it mean the child is brain-damaged? Will difficult diets be necessary? When will it end? And meanwhile how do you cope?

The terms used to describe hyperactivity are rather confusing, especially as American definitions of hyperactivity tend to differ from British ones. British child psychiatrists make the diagnosis 'hyperkinetic disorder' if a child is extremely restless and inattentive in a variety of situations; often there are signs of slow development, like poor co-ordination or delayed speech. In fact such symptoms were sometimes termed 'minimal brain damage' because of the number of minor neurological abnormalities.

Parents generally use the word hyperactivity to cover symptoms which include a high activity level, an apparent lack of need for sleep, impulsiveness, taking risks, poor self-control, poor concentration, defiance and disobedience. All this behaviour is unfortunately common in small boys, but this does not mean it is easy to deal with.

Some parents wonder if their child's hyperactivity is a sign of high intelligence with a restless, unsatisfied curiosity which may need a different educational approach. Sometimes, children's concentration is so poor that their parents are concerned that they may be suffering from food allergies, especially to additives; the evidence on this issue is mixed.

Hyperactivity is sometimes offered as a label by schools rather than parents, usually for a child who concentrates poorly, does not stay in his seat, may even run out of school and also is generally disruptive and even aggressive.

Modern research emphasises the need to look at the details of the hyperactivity. How much is it a behaviour problem? Is it mainly a concentration problem? Is there underlying anxiety or depression? These questions are particularly relevant when the use of medication is being considered.

Case histories

Andrew, aged 8, was brought to the child guidance clinic by his mother because of his very poor attention and strange behaviour in school. He seemed to be an unusually anxious rather than a naughty child, but his mother felt that she should exclude dietary factors before looking at any psychological issues and was therefore referred on to a children's hospital that was carrying out research into the effects of diet on behaviour.

A year later she returned with Andrew. There did seem to be some connection between Andrew's most difficult times and particular foods, so some improvement had been gained by reducing his intake of these. However, there were still considerable problems at school and these were gradually sorted out with psychotherapy for Andrew, advice to his mother and the provision of special education.

◆

Ben had always seemed very alert as a baby, slept poorly and was easily upset. As a toddler, his speech was advanced, he always wanted new entertainments and was easily frustrated, leading to temper tantrums. He immediately mastered the 'child-proof' medicine cabinet and handed out pills to his friends. He was exhausting for his parents and play-group organisers. At a more formally structured nursery school, his energies were organised and his 'brightness' became an asset rather than a drawback.

◆

Janet was referred to the child guidance unit aged 10 because of difficult behaviour, poor concentration and poor attainment. Her school and her mother thought Janet was hyperactive but her father thought she did not have any problems.

During the interview Janet's low opinion of herself and her unhappiness at school became clear. Detailed psychological assessment showed that in her case she was if anything over-achieving in terms of reading but was actually quite developmentally immature in several respects, and finding it difficult to cope in an ordinary school.

Janet and her family were seen regularly for support by the clinic and arrangements were made for special educational support. Even before this was available, a calmer and more structured approach, as school, family and clinic worked together, resulted in considerable improvement of Janet's behaviour and consequently of her relationship with her school.

What parents can do

If the main problems of hyperactivity are at home, try to work out in detail what they consist of and discuss with other parents how they manage similar problems. You may find that your child is much more difficult at certain times of day – such as before school or with one parent rather than the other. If so this may be a clue to when to give extra attention and also when to 'take a deep breath' yourself, so as not to worsen the situation by losing your cool.

Some young children seem unable to relax, won't take a midday rest and get more and more demanding in the evenings. Though proud of your own child's thirst for stimulation and information, remember that you all need rest and a break from each other sometimes. So be firm about bedtimes so that your child gets enough sleep.

If you begin to think that your child's overactivity, concentration difficulties or fractiousness may be related to food, then consult your health visitor, clinic doctor or GP. It is very sensible to ensure that your child has a good diet and there may be one or two things which upset him – too many caffeinated fizzy drinks (such as colas) in particular may be bad for the nerves as well as bad for the teeth.

If you want to take it further, a dietitian or paediatric specialist would be the right person. Beware of extreme diets to remedy hypothetical allergies, as these may cause other nutritional problems.

If the hyperactivity and poor concentration is mainly a problem at school do try to find out all details calmly, as behaviour at school can sometimes be amazingly different from that at home. In order to intervene, it is very important to know about the child's ability, attainments and the demands being put on him. Do not just accept impressions, but ask for an assessment by an educational psychologist. The child may have good ability, for instance, but because of concentration difficulties may have poor reading skills and be trying to cover this up by distracting and disruptive behaviour. (See also Chapter 7.)

Medication is occasionally worth trying for children with hyperactivity, but this decision is best made by a specialist child psychiatric centre rather than a GP. Tranquillisers are rarely appropriate; but stimulant and antidepressant type drugs have been shown to have some effectiveness although they do not make much difference in the long term.

Useful organisations

Hyperactive Children's Support Group
    71 Whyte Lane
    Chichester
    Sussex
    Tel: 0903 725182
Provides help and information to families with hyperactive children.

The Institute of Psychiatry
    De Crespigny Park Road
    London SE5
    Tel: 071 703 5411
Specialist centre for the assessment and treatment of hyperactive children.

IS MY CHILD SCHIZOPHRENIC?

Schizophrenia

'I think my son must be schizophrenic' announced the mother of a seven-year-old who on some days could be charming and on other days violently bad-tempered. But the term schizophrenia is not just a general description of anyone whose personality seems to vary greatly from time to time. Schizophrenia, although still not well understood, is an illness which can have a very poor outcome, in which the normal boundaries between fantasy and reality become weakened. A sufferer typically becomes convinced that the television news is particularly directed at him and that he can hear neighbours discussing him critically or even plotting against him. This sort of experience can be intensely distressing and can lead to outbursts of (to outsiders) incomprehensible aggression, or to attempts at suicide.

The first things relatives might notice may be increasing social withdrawal, preoccupation with certain themes – such as the supernatural – suspiciousness and irritability and a loss of interest in the tasks of daily life including self-care.

Such symptoms are extremely rare before puberty, but the illness itself is quite common, affecting about eight in 1,000 of the population. However, schizophrenia often starts in the teenage years, so it is important not to dismiss early signs as normal adolescent truculence, although sometimes the distinction is hard to make.

Case histories

Ellen was referred as an emergency to the child guidance unit by her school. She was 14 and for the previous few weeks had been reluctant to go to school, had begun talking of incidents out of books as if they were real, seemed to be seeing someone 'in white' and was afraid of being burned and dying.

At school that day she had been mumbling and making no sense, saying the children were laughing at her, then laughing and rocking and picking things off her sleeve which were not there.

When seen at the clinic she mostly looked away and giggled inappropriately. She then became suddenly angry at the questions and said she was 'not saying ... on tape ... in the past'. No real communication was possible as she appeared to be distracted by her own thoughts.

Ellen's previous personality had been quiet, but otherwise normal. She had not undergone any serious recent stresses. She may have had a genetic vulnerability however, as it was known her father had been admitted to a mental hospital on several occasions.

Ellen was quickly admitted to a psychiatric in-patient unit for adolescents where she remained for several months. Her illness responded well to the appropriate medication and she was able to return to school. Later, she became ill again, though less severely, and returned for treatment. She is now successfully living independently of her family, remaining under psychiatric review.

◆

Jacob, aged 13, was also admitted to the adolescent psychiatric unit. At school he had become very withdrawn, hid behind cupboards and had lost interest in everything except reading the Bible.

At home he was irritable with his mother, shouted at her and refused to eat food she had prepared. Sometimes he would talk non-stop. At the interview with the doctor he was smiling to himself, saying occasional words and seemed quite cut off from what was happening around him.

Jacob had been known to the child guidance unit when he was younger – the problems at that time were of poor reading and disobedience at home. His mother suffered intermittently from mental illness herself which added to the difficulties of caring for this very sick boy.

Jacob went on to a special boarding school, which was very helpful for two years, but when Jacob started to wander off naked he was expelled and subsequently was taken into care by social services.

◆

Della, 15, became convinced that the girls at school were bullying her and trying to poison her and started to refuse to go, becoming also generally defiant and difficult with her parents. It turned out that she was a somewhat over-protected only child and indeed much adored only grand-daughter.

She had a moderately low level of ability, as revealed by developmental tests when younger. This had been masked by excellent teaching and supportive parents. However, as Della approached 16, her feelings of being different from the other girls and her fear of failing the exams ahead increased, and she was in fact quite depressed. Anti-depressant treatment started by the GP was very helpful, and further treatment by the child psychiatry department consisted of support for both the girl and her family and negotiations with the school to reduce the demands of the curriculum.

What parents can do

Although all three teenagers above had severe symptoms, only the first two were diagnosed as having schizophrenia. This conclusion is never arrived at rapidly and there is no simple test that can immediately reveal the condition. This means that there may be months, even years, of uncertainty.

Usually, suspected cases are treated by initial hospitalisation for assessment and the start of medication. Sometimes there is a rapid and permanent recovery; for others, long-term follow-up and treatment by mental health services will be necessary. Parents may find extreme difficulties getting appropriate help for children like this, especially when the child becomes a young adult, but has no insight into the need for care when he or she is ill. Matters are not helped for you as parents, either, if you are made to feel blamed for the illness, or told that schizophrenia is not a 'real' illness anyway. All these factors tend to influence the poor provision of resources, and it can be par ticularly difficult to achieve a smooth transition from children's to adult provision of care.

However, schizophrenia is a condition that can be helped, and research shows that families can contribute greatly to this if they are advised and supported. Make sure that your child sees your GP and is referred on to a child psychiatric service that is used to dealing with adolescents.

Useful organisations

MIND (National Association for Mental Health)
22 Harley Street
London W1N 2ED
Tel: 071 637 0741
Information and advice service.

National Schizophrenia Fellowship
28 Castle Street
Kingston-upon-Thames
Surrey KT1 1SS
Tel: 081 547 3937
Provides advice service; sets up regional self-help groups for relatives of those with schizophrenia.

The Richmond Fellowship (for Community Mental Health)
8 Addison Road
London W14 8DL
Tel: 071 603 6373

IS MY CHILD SCHOOL PHOBIC?

School phobia

In adult psychiatric terms a phobia is a fear, often quite specific, which is recognised as irrational by the sufferer who wants to be able to overcome it and resume a normal life. 'School phobia' is much more complex. The classic case is of a child who has fairly recently started secondary school and begins to develop tummy-aches on the mornings of school days, perhaps especially on one particular day of the week. If allowed to stay at home the symptoms pass off, but anxiety may be evident in the evening at the thought of school the next day. The following morning, if put under pressure to attend, the child seems white and shaky, may even vomit and angrily resists the idea of going to school.

What is the cause? Most children, if asked what they don't like about their school, will tell you in considerable detail. In contrast some school phobic children will say something fairly general such as that they don't like the teachers or the children; others will just say 'nothing' or 'don't know'. It is thus peculiarly difficult to find out what is bothering the child and little in the way of a single precipitating incident or trauma may ever be discovered. Nevertheless it is clear that change of school can be a factor; so can other pressures such as bullying or difficulties in coping with academic demands.

Often the situation at home is the key. The school phobic child is frequently the youngest child of older parents who may, for some reason such as illness in babyhood or the death of another relative, have been particularly protected by his or her parents. Sometimes one of the parents has a severe illness such as asthma or epilepsy. These situations lead to understandable separation anxiety, so that the major fear is of being away from the parents (usually the mother), rather than of being present at school. An anxious child like this often tells a psychiatrist or psychologist that he or she is worrying about mother being run over, but the parent may have no idea of this.

A child who is playing truant, rather than a school phobic, openly dislikes school, is often not doing well academically and is usually out of the house with a group of like-minded friends. It may be quite a while before the parents even realise what is happening, as notices from the school may be intercepted and 'sick-notes' forged.

Case histories

Carole stopped attending her secondary school after only a few weeks, saying that the girls picked on her. She had also become generally unhappy and withdrawn and would not even mix with friends and family.

She was the youngest of 13 children, others of whom had been truants. She was an inarticulate girl, of limited academic ability, so that one could see that ordinary secondary school life might have been quite difficult. In addition, it turned out that her father had just died unexpectedly and her mother, who not unnaturally became quite depressed, brought her in to sleep with her at night. This family needed considerable support from the combined efforts of the educational welfare service, the school psychological service and the child psychiatry department. Carole eventually settled successfully at a special school for 'delicate' children which was able to offer a less demanding environment and curriculum than an ordinary secondary school.

◆

Paul's morning tummy-aches were so bad that he was brought into hospital for investigation. He also had only just started secondary school and his troubles seemed to start after a fall from his bike.

He was the youngest of two boys, separated by some

years, and it later emerged that there had been a still-birth in between.

After considering the options Paul's mother and father decided that they did want help to return Paul to his usual school and met with the child psychiatrist at the school to work out how to do this. Luckily there was a small support unit within the school with an experienced teacher who was prepared to withstand Paul's tantrums, and a programme of gradual reassimilation into the ordinary classroom day was introduced.

Paul remained anxious about break, assembly and games, but his general confidence increased and he was able to do well academically.

◆

Terry, aged 14, was referred to the clinic by the educational welfare service. He had been attending school very poorly for the previous two terms, sometimes arriving but bunking off later. When out of school he was usually with friends, and had been recently picked up by the police for shop-lifting.

He was the second of two boys and lived with his father, step-mother and her two children. Academically he tended to fool around when he was in class and could have achieved more.

Some help was given to the family at the clinic, and the educational welfare officer worked with the school to offer Terry a place in the school support unit, which Terry much preferred and attended far more.

What parents can do

An occasional example of this kind of school anxiety

not uncommon with younger children, particularly after illness, and can be overcome by kind but firm handling and co-operation between home and school.

However, although school phobic children are certainly anxious and sometimes depressed too, they can be very irritating children to deal with, so not all schools can offer the right mixture of flexibility and firm encouragement. Parents must take an active role to achieve success and professional back-up and guidance is useful. There are a variety of treatment approaches offered for school phobia, with family therapy and behavioural therapy being probably most successful in achieving a return to school. The education social work service is likely to be involved if the non-attendance is considerable, and can provide support and referral to appropriate agencies.

Parents will be wondering if they should insist on their child going to school – perhaps the pressure is too great? They should take their time in considering this and sometimes a less pressured school environment does turn out to be the solution.

Difficulties may also occur if the parents cannot muster sufficient resources to help the distressed child overcome his or her insecurity. This happens particularly if, for instance, a divorced mother feels insufficiently supported by her ex-husband, or if the parents actually do not think the particular school – or even the entire educational system – is right for their child.

Recommendations for hospital admission, boarding school and home tuition are less usual nowadays. What they have in common is that they bring the education to the child rather than the child to the education and so can fail to resolve underlying issues. This may lead to problems in adult life, as avoiding difficulties instead of facing them is 'learned' as the best way to manage.

Useful organisations

Education Otherwise
  25 Common Lane
  Hemmingford Abbots
  Cambridgeshire
  Tel: 0480 63130
Helps those who wish to educate their children at home.

Phobic Action
  Greater London House
  547–551 High Road
  Leytonstone
  London E11 4PR
  Tel: 081 558 6012

6

BODY OR MIND?

The mind and body affect each other with children, just as with adults, though the results of this sometimes take different forms. Poor hearing, for instance, might not seem to be linked to behaviour problems yet this can be the case. In the opposite direction, stress and worry can cause physical symptoms such as headaches or bed-wetting. This chapter looks at some of these links.

HEARING AND SIGHT

Major handicaps of sight and of hearing are usually quite obvious to parents and are picked up by the developmental screening provided at the health clinic or by your GP. However, when problems are minor, intermittent or develop gradually they are more difficult to detect, and sometimes the underlying difficulty may be missed for quite a while.

Hearing

It was once said that a notice saying 'Can this child hear?' should be hung on the back of every child psychiatrist's door – and this was wise advice.

Glue ear (the result of chronic ear infections) is surprisingly common in young children and can lead to bouts of partial hearing loss or even complete deafness. This may not be recognised by parents or diagnosed by medical staff – and it is quite difficult to test the hearing of a fidgety child.

A child who has not heard cannot of course obey – so sometimes behaviour problems seem to be the main difficulty. And children who have had intermittent poor hearing may be slow to speak as a result. This can lead to frustration in expressing themselves and temper tantrums.

Children who have suffered in the past from occasional deafness sometimes seem to have learned to 'tune out' requests, even when they can hear, and may need a lot of help in settling into the demands of school life. The bustling sounds of a modern infant classroom and the lack of clear visual signs to act as a guide can also prove confusing. Such children may very quickly earn labels such as 'distractable', 'disobedient' and 'disruptive'.

◆

Jason, for instance, was referred to the clinic by his school at the age of six when he was still in the infants class. His behaviour was very difficult as he never seemed to sit still, never listened and never did what he was told. Although he seemed to be averagely bright he was making very little progress in learning to read and write. Jason was certainly inattentive and when observed in his open-plan classroom he just buzzed around, gaining attention by mischievousness rather than settling to work. His speaking skills were poor and when his mother was asked about his development it turned out that his speech had been delayed at the age of three and that hearing tests had shown that he was moderately deaf, especially in one ear. Grommets (a kind of drainage tube) had been inserted in his ears and this had led to some improvement of his speech, hearing and attention. However, the after-effects were still evident, even now that Jason no longer had a hearing problem.

So, if you think your child may have a hearing difficulty make absolutely sure that he or she is tested by the most up-to-date methods in the best possible conditions – and if there is any doubt have him or her tested again. Go to your clinic, school doctor or GP to arrange this.

Vision

Undiagnosed visual problems are more likely to lead to unexplained educational failure than behaviour problems. Again, eye problems are usually picked up through routine clinic or school testing, but some children can slip through the net so it is worth checking if you have any worries about their eyes.

Occasionally quite subtle problems of eye co-ordination can be the cause of apparent dyslexia.

Useful organisations

National Deaf Children's Society
   45 Hereford Road
   London W2 5AH
   Tel: 071 229 9272
Provides a self-help support service.

WORRIES CAUSING PHYSICAL SYMPTOMS

Sometimes it is clear to everybody that some sort of worry is probably the cause of a physical symptom, for instance the tummy-ache every Monday morning before the games lesson. Even though the symptoms may be severe and accompanied by paleness, sweating and vomiting or diarrhoea, the timing – usually in the morning – and the duration – usually in relation to a feared event – give clues.

Sometimes 'emotional' tummy-aches are referred to as abdominal migraine and indeed some of these children do grow up to have adult-type tension headaches or migraine.

Most families recognise a child's susceptibility towards certain physical symptoms and learn to act appropriately but there are times when a child has, say, persistent head aches or abdominal pain and seems so distressed that re assurance from the GP is not enough. This may happen particularly if your faith in the medical profession has been undermined by, for instance, some previous failure to diagnose a serious condition. In these circumstances you may be irritated or upset by a suggestion that your child be referred to someone like a child psychiatrist and you may want to get a more specialist opinion from a paediatrician first. However, a child can act as a lightning conductor for unhappiness or tension within a family, and tummy-aches, headaches or 'growing pains', although very real to the sufferer, can nevertheless have their origins in stresses such as marriage difficulties or the death of a grandparent.

Aisha, for instance, aged nine, was the youngest child of four and was having repeated tummy-aches. They were fairly clearly associated with anxiety as she was also having nightmares and had various fears of school such as of a ghost in the tower.

The family had a number of stresses, including several deaths amongst the extended family. The mother had taken up child-minding to supplement the family finances and it seemed that Aisha was feeling rather displaced.

Treatment of such a situation, whether through family or individual therapy, may not uncover a single clear cause but allowing anxieties to be aired and improving family communication can often help. Sometimes psychosomatic symptoms are clearly related to a specific past trauma.

Gregory, aged 10, also had morning tummy-aches, which felt like 'a man inside trying to get out'. Although most of the time he seemed confident and assertive, he became very anxious at night, finding it difficult to get off to sleep and also could not make progress in learning to read. He was an only child living with his divorced mother. One night, two years previously, his mother's ex-boyfriend had come to the house, chloroformed Gregory and kidnapped his mother. Later, in prison, the boyfriend killed himself.

Gregory was seen individually by the child psychiatrist at the child guidance unit, while his mother saw the psychiatric social worker, and over several months the symptoms began to decline.

Occasionally, children develop more unusual physical symptoms which, after investigation, do not seem to have a physical basis and may even be described as being 'hysterical'.

Janine, aged 12, developed a persistent sneeze which lasted for several months. Paediatric investigations proved negative but there was no improvement and the problem was interfering with Janine's education as she was being sent out of class if she had a sneezing fit.

The family were seen by the child psychiatric department but the mother still felt that something was being overlooked from the medical point of view – just as had happened when her older brother had undiagnosed heart problems and had died suddenly.

Although they had to acknowledge a difference in views, the family and the therapists were able to work together on ideas as to how to manage the problem to cause less upset – whatever the cause – and the sneezing stopped fairly quickly.

———————◆———————

Tessa developed a dragging of her foot which her mother was naturally very worried about. Paediatric assessment revealed no physical cause, so Tessa was referred on to the child psychiatry department where she was seen with her mother and sister.

Her parents were divorced and the mother had a developing relationship with a new boyfriend. Tessa was the elder of two girls and was compared unfavourably with the younger one who was considered by the family to be prettier and to have a more out-going and pleasant personality. Listening to everybody's concerns in detail and helping the family to communicate with each other provided sufficient support and help for improvement in two interviews.

So if your child develops a symptom which the GP, the paediatrician and yourselves think may have an emotional basis, then it is worth getting appropriate specialist help. Usually this sort of psychosomatic problem resolves itself over a few months.

AFTER ILLNESS

Often after a viral illness such a flu or glandular fever physical symptoms seem to linger on, perhaps in the form of tiring easily and loss of interest and energy. Sometimes emotional symptoms predominate, such as irritability, tearfulness, wanting to withdraw socially and being anxious about school.

Some of these cases would nowadays be considered to be myalgic encephalomyelitis (ME) which is also now referred to as chronic fatigue syndrome. Not all doctors believe that this is a disease in itself, but most accept that when there has been an original illness a child may need time for rehabilitation for both physical and emotional after-effects.

Stuart had suffered a severe flu-like illness at the age of 11, in the year following his father's sudden death from a heart attack. At 14, he was referred to the child psychiatrist by his school, who were concerned at his apathy and listlessness and wondered if he was depressed. Stuart agreed he tired easily but he did still have enough energy and interest to run his own rock group. He denied any unhappiness, although it was clear that there were points of tension with his mother.

On the whole his physical and mental state seemed to be gradually improving together, and although mother and son were convinced that the father's death was irrelevant to the problem, some short-term psychological support was accepted and steady progress continued.

◆

Carla had always been a bright, energetic and hardworking little girl who enjoyed school and life in general. She became quite ill and encephalomyelitis (a viral disease of the nervous system) was diagnosed. The recovery period was very prolonged, so that even after 18 months had passed she was reluctant to return to school. When her parents more or less forced her to attend school, she became exhausted and upset – but medically there were no signs of actual illness. The parents were not aware of any other family stresses and were very puzzled as to how to handle Carla – not knowing whether to insist on school attendance or to continue to make allowances.

In the end gentle persistence by her parents paid off, with support from the paediatrician, the child psychiatrist and the school. Carla joined a younger class at school and her time-table was modified so that she could pace her re-entry comfortably.

Useful organisations

ME Association
   Stanhope House
   High Street
   Stanhope-le-Hope
   Essex SS17 0HA
   Tel: 0375 642466

IN HOSPITAL FOR AN OPERATION

Hospitals used to be very frightening places for children, and parents' visits were highly restricted because they seemed to cause more distress and prevent the child from settling down.

It was eventually realised that even though to the nurses

and doctors on the ward the children did not seem to be disturbed by their experience, the small patients were often going home with many symptoms of unhappiness and anxiety such as clinging and bed-wetting. Research also showed that sometimes the effects were quite severe and prolonged.

Hospitals usually manage to be efficient and caring places, so what is it about them that makes admission to hospital so stressful? First, the illness itself – such as appendicitis – may be very sudden and painful, and the whole family may be extremely concerned until the diagnosis is clear and until everyone is sure that the child will safely recover.

Even if the operation is a planned one – such as a squint repair or a circumcision – the young child may not really understand what will happen and may worry that the particular part of his body may be damaged or out of action for ever.

Then the treatments themselves may be frightening and painful – injections and blood tests, for instance – as well as the after-effects of an operation. Loss of the ability to move around, for example after leg or back operations, can also be frustrating and depressing.

But perhaps the greatest strain for children is not merely their helplessness in a strange environment, but the loss of their normal home comforts and the protective company of their parents.

Flora and Dean were both two-year-olds and were observed over the days that they were in hospital for an operation to correct their squints. At first both were normal bouncy two-year-olds, chatty in their own ways and interested in new things and people. Flora was lucky enough to be able to have her mother stay with her all the time and seemed little affected by the operation. Dean's mother, however, could not be with him so much and after the operation he became quite withdrawn and would not engage in chat or play.

◆

Harry was referred to the clinic at seven because of his anxiety and poor concentration at school. When he was five he had an operation to bring one testicle down, and though this is a small operation, for Harry it had been a major and frightening event which he had not fully understood. Because something 'bad' had happened to him, he felt he must have done something wrong and was being punished – but he could not tell anyone.

Fortunately, the family stresses which had made it difficult for his parents to give Harry sufficient loving support over the time of his operation had now passed, and Harry soon began to improve with therapy from the clinic and some extra help at school.

Teenagers, too, sometimes fail to cope with a hospital admission as well as might be expected. Often hospitals do not have a separate adolescent ward but environments geared to younger children or to adults are not appropriate. Adolescents need the company of others of their own age group to compare notes and make friendships. And ward staff also need special skills of the right mix of making allowances but being firm.

Cheryl, aged 14, needed a back operation because of an infection in her spine. She was admitted first to an adult ward and later to a children's ward. Neither ward was used to dealing much with adolescents and Cheryl's recovery took a stormy course which seemed to be more related to emotional than physical factors, though with pain this can be a very difficult distinction to make. Cheryl's parents at times felt they were not being told everything, but on the other hand the ward staff were a little frightened of them because they expressed themselves in such a forthright way.

Cheryl was not one to confide her feelings much, but it seemed likely that this physical set-back was affecting her in the one particular area she excelled at – athletics. Meanwhile her parents were also coping with the grief of a bereavement; the grandmother who was 'the backbone of the family' had just died.

A social worker and child psychiatrist met several times with the family, talked to Cheryl on her own and worked jointly with the nurses and the physiotherapist to help Cheryl become confident enough to walk again.

You can reduce the stress of a child's admission by preparation beforehand:

- Inform yourself as much as possible about what to expect and arrange to take the child along to the ward before the admission to meet some of the staff and see the layout.
- Ask if you can stay, as with an under-five the presence of the mother or father is the greatest reassurance.
- Ensure as much continuity and familiarity for the small child as possible. This means bringing along teddy and the favourite blanket, books and tapes and family photographs.
- Tell the staff about your child's normal routine and what might especially distress or comfort them if you are not there.
- Do what you can to explain to your child what is going to happen to their body in the operation. It may be best to do this with one of the members of staff, using toys and drawing. Imagine being in the child's

place and not knowing what a squint operation, or a circumcision, might involve.

After the operation, either in the hospital or at home, there may still be signs of unhappiness or anxiety sometimes coming out as naughtiness, so be prepared to talk thing over again and make allowances for a while.

Wards are much happier places for children these days and play staff and teaching staff particularly contribute to this and are always pleased to talk to parents.

Useful organisations

The Hospital's 'League of Friends'

Action for Sick Children (The National Association for the Welfare of Children in Hospital)
Argyle House
29–31 Euston Road
London NW1 2SD
Tel: 071 833 2041
Advises families and campaigns for improved standards of care for children in hospital.

LONG-TERM INTERMITTENT ILLNESS

Parents with children who suffer from relatively common but sometimes seriously disabling conditions such as asthma, eczema, diabetes, epilepsy or blood disorders such as sickle cell disease or haemophilia, may well find that these conditions are made worse by stress.

This is of course not the same as being *caused* by stress and if your child is referred to someone from the child psychiatry or psychology department it is usually because they often work with the child's paediatrician and know quite a lot about the particular type of illness and its effect on families and children. It does not mean that the illness is thought to be imaginary in any way, or the fault of the parents.

Tony, as a baby, had several fits caused by fever, which required admission to hospital. He was put on anticonvulsant medication until the age of five, when it was withdrawn because he was fit-free. He had never been an easy child and there were also lots of family problems, so when two years later he began to have severe nightmares and also tempers followed by exhaustion, it was hard to tell whether these were fit-related or not. A combined approach from the paediatrician and the child psychiatry department in the hospital turned out to be the best way of managing the problem. This was happily accepted by the mother when she realised that it was not a case of purely body *or* mind.

———————— ◆ ————————

Georgina, aged six, had severe asthmatic attacks which meant that she had to go into hospital on an emergency basis, sometimes in the middle of the night. Her mother had become worn out and distressed by this and the behaviour of the two older children became very difficult. The father was spending more and more time outside the home on committee work.

During one of Georgina's hospital admissions the ward staff thought that the staff from the child psychiatry department might be able to help and so a psychiatric social worker and a child psychiatrist arranged to meet the whole family. It was clear that the family was in a sort of vicious circle of stress, which seemed to contribute to making the asthma worse.

The family welcomed the opportunity to reflect on the situation once they realised that it was not a question of blame and began to think together of ways to handle things better. The older children had pertinent observations to make about how Georgina always got her own way, and the mother began to think about how she could organise time just for herself and perhaps even return to work. The father was criticised by his family in the first session, but coped with this, and kept coming.

After six family sessions the atmosphere was much better, and it seemed that problems were more easily sorted out. Georgina's night crises had also reduced, though she continued to need her regular anti-asthmatic medication.

───────── ◆ ─────────

Lorraine, aged six, had extremely severe eczema over much of her skin and had been referred because of increasing unhappiness about going to school where she had few friends. She had missed quite a bit of school anyway because of her illness and was therefore at risk of falling behind. When she was under stress, she tended to scratch more, so it looked as if a vicious circle was developing.

At home, Lorraine was the third of four children, but there were no major problems. On contacting the school, however, it emerged that some of the teachers thought that Lorraine's skin condition was so severe that she should not be attending ordinary school at all, because of the unsightliness and possible risk to herself.

The best help for this situation was thought to be the school nurse and school doctor who could advise on making appropriate allowances for Lorraine, while at the same time encouraging her to take as full a part in school life as possible. Fortunately, the headmistress lent her authority to this approach and Lorraine began to settle down.

◆

Leroy, aged 11, had sickle cell disease – an illness to which people of African origin may be genetically susceptible. In winter, especially if he had a cold or flu, he was likely to need admission for 'sickle cell crises', when the blood cells in his body stuck together causing a lot of pain. His mother knew the problem well and had other relatives with the same illness. However, not all the casualty doctors and at first not Leroy's school were as understanding or as knowledgeable. It became clear to the specialist sickle cell clinic that, for the children attending to do as well as possible, it was important also to have an educational function for the hospital staff and the community at large, and also to provide a counselling service for the families. With these extra staff, the clinic was able to help Leroy's mother to communicate with his school about his falling behind because of the illness and sort out how to help him catch up again.

f your child is attending a paediatric clinic over a long period, you might like to consider asking whether any psychological help of any kind is available, especially if you are aware that stress may be making your child's illness worse. There is now evidence that family therapy, or instance, can help in the management and control of childhood asthma and diabetes.

Useful organisations

British Diabetic Association
  10 Queen Anne Street
  London W1M OBD
  Tel: 071 323 1531
Provides practical help and advice.

British Epilepsy Association
  Anstey House
  40 Hanover Square
  Leeds LS3 1BE
  Tel: 0532 439393
Provides practical advice and support.

Haemophilia Society
  123 Westminster Bridge Road
  London SE1 7HR
  Tel: 071 928 2020
Helps and advises those with haemophilia and their relatives.

National Asthma Campaign
  Providence House
  Providence Place
  London N1 0NT
  Tel: 071 226 2260
Provides information and help for those with asthma and their families.

National Eczema Society
  4 Tavistock Place
  London WC1H 9RA
  Tel: 071 388 4097
Provides information and advice for those with eczema and to their families.

National Society for Epilepsy
   Chalfont Centre for Epilepsy
   Chalfont St Peter
   Buckinghamshire
   Tel: 02407 3991

Sickle Cell Society
   54 Station Road North
   London NW10 4UA
   Tel: 081 961 4006
Provides help, information and support to families affected by sickle cell disease through home and hospital visits, plus financial help when necessary.

THE HANDICAPPED CHILD

At first parents may find it hard to believe they have produced a handicapped child and may become angry or feel guilty as they look for answers to the unanswerable question – 'Why us?' Later parents sometimes describe how they had to go through a process of mourning and grieving for the healthy child they did not have.

Different families react differently to such a major stress – which can pose an economic as well as an emotional burden. For some parents it may be become a final straw in an unhappy relationship. Others may find themselves working together to overcome the handicap, or to look for the best possible information and treatment.

The wider family also has mixed emotions when faced with a handicapped addition to a family. Some may become less involved than previously. Older children are likely to try to be helpful and caring, but may sometimes feel their own needs are being overlooked in the process.

The handicapped child himself or herself may be protected very much by the family environment at first, but later find themselves subject to misunderstanding, teasing and social rejection, depending on the nature of the disability.

Ellen was born very prematurely and was diagnosed as suffering from cerebral palsy. However, by the age of eight the obvious physical signs were no longer evident. She was attending a special school for delicate children, but had few friends and often had temper tantrums with screaming for no apparent reason. She found difficulty in physical sequences, such as putting on a cardigan, and it was difficult to follow her train of thought in conversation. Ellen's academic abilities were below average, although her vocabulary was good. At home she tended to be teased by her three brothers and defended and protected by her parents, especially her mother. At this stage advice to the school was offered and a more detailed assessment by the educational psychologist was arranged.

When Ellen was referred again at the age of 14, she had no obvious physical problems but seemed immature and was still finding it difficult to make friends. Her mother was very worried about her; suppose she allowed her out unaccompanied, as the teachers were suggesting – what if a stranger took advantage of her? And what could she do when she left school? Ellen herself was sad because she wanted to have nice clothes and have boyfriends and felt she was unattractive.

Fortunately the school became more aware of Ellen's emotional neediness in negotiating adolescence and were able to provide counselling by a teacher.

◆

Lynette was also seen by the child psychiatrist over a prolonged period. She had very poor vision, found school work extremely difficult as she had a moderate mental handicap and was already at a special school. Her behaviour was difficult too, and when frustrated she tended to pick at her skin. Her mother, and indeed her teachers, found her extremely irritating but telling her off simply made her worse.

By the age of 15 Lynette was a very fat and unhappy girl and prone to arguing with people. She still had her own normal adolescent wishes and longed one day to have her independence, a flat, a husband and a baby. She thought it was not fair that just because she was handicapped she was not allowed out by herself.

It is well known that some handicaps are more acceptable socially than others, even though life is still far from easy for the sufferers. For instance, a child who is obviously blind or is in a wheel-chair but otherwise looks 'normal' and can converse and behave reasonably well usually evokes sympathy and helpfulness. But a child who looks a bit unusual, and who may behave unpredictably because of a variety of physical impairments can evoke rejection, which is likely to exacerbate any emotional disturbance. Parents may be very stressed by the effort of making allowances and special arrangements and cannot, as with a fully normal child, look confidently forward to the day when the child will grow to safe adulthood and independence. They are often rightly concerned about the particular dangers of sexual abuse of handicapped young people.

Self-help groups certainly have their place, so that parents can discover they are not alone with their difficulties. Yet just because the emotional strain on parents and children is understandable, this does not mean that extra psychological help cannot sometimes be appropriate. This can sometimes be provided by social workers or psychologists attached to special schools who have built up expertise in the particular type of handicap – such as epilepsy or autism. These professionals will also usually know about the local child psychiatric services if further help seems advisable.

Useful organisations

Contact a Family
    16 Strutton Ground
    London SW1P 2HP
    Tel: 071 222 2695
A link service for families who have a physically and/or mentally handicapped child, so they can share help and support.

Down's Syndrome Association
    155 Mitcham Road
    London SW17 9PG
    Tel: 081 682 4001
Gives practical support, advice and information.

Kids
    80 Waynflete Square
    London W10 6UD
    Tel: 081 969 2817
Works with parents to help children with developmental or learning problems or who have a mental or physical disability.

Royal Society for Mentally Handicapped Children and
    Adults (MENCAP)
    Mencap National Centre
    123 Golden Lane
    London EC1Y ORT
    Tel: 071 454 0454

Spastics Society
    12 Park Crescent
    London W1N 4EQ
    Tel: 071 636 5020
Advice and information for parents of children with
cerebral palsy. Call free – Cerebral Palsy Helpline – 0800
626216.

LIFE-THREATENING ILLNESS

While, these days, very severe illnesses are rare in children,
they can of course have a devastating emotional effect on
the child him or herself, the parents and rest of the family.
Cystic fibrosis, leukaemia and liver or kidney disease are
examples of childhood conditions which used to bring an
early death but now can be helped considerably – sometimes even cured. However, not merely is the illness frightening, painful or disfiguring, but the medical and surgical
treatments themselves can be very distressing and sometimes necessitate frequent or long hospital admissions at
specialist centres miles from home. The prolonged uncertainty about the outcome is also very stressful, and it is
very hard for parents to work out how much they should
insist on 'normal' standards of behaviour with a child who
is sometimes very sick.

Leo, aged 12, had leukaemia and began to be very
difficult about accepting further courses of treatment.
For him, one of the most distressing aspects was that
his hair had all fallen out, so that even when he was
well enough to go to school he was very reluctant to do
so. His mother and father were split about how to
handle this crisis, as were the professionals who themselves were becoming uncertain about the benefits of
any treatment.

A social worker and child psychotherapist met the family and began to help them to sort out some of their painful and difficult feelings, and to decide together what would be the best for Leo given that the treatment was so unpleasant and painful, and the returns seemed to be possibly diminishing.

Under these sorts of serious but uncertain conditions, parents may be surprised to find how angry they feel as well as distressed, and possibly guilty and afraid. These natural negative emotions surface in lots of different ways; sometimes in searching for someone or something to blame parents may get angry with each other. Or in trying to avoid the pain, parents become more distant from each other.

Some parents become very involved in and knowledgeable about their child's medical condition, others find the situation so distressing that they begin to avoid coming to the hospital ward much at all. The sound of the telephone ringing is alarming because of the possible bad news; approaching the ward brings on fear of what they might be about to see or hear.

Elizabeth was born unexpectedly early and consequently had a very low birth weight. She was being looked after in the intensive care baby unit. She was having frequent crises and each time it seemed that she might die. Even if she survived her chance of being handicapped later was increased. The staff noticed that Elizabeth's mother was very anxious when she came on to the ward, and had begun to come in less often. After the mother herself had left hospital she had quite a long journey to return, and also had another daughter of four at home.

The liaison health visitor got to know the mother

well, and encouraged her to visit bringing her husband and other daughter too. They planned the discharge date together as Elizabeth's condition became more stable, and both parents and the grandmother learned the procedures to help Elizabeth feed properly.

Although the time of taking her home was still full of anxiety, the good trust and communication developed between the ward and the parents helped to overcome the small problems that did arise.

Some specialist units have their own counsellors, often nurse-counsellors, who know about the nature of the illness as well as having had counselling training. Sometimes the hospital social worker may be able to offer regular counselling help, run parent groups and generally be available for advice. Sometimes the hospital chaplain has a special role in offering support on the paediatric wards.

Medical and nursing staff also feel the strain, but try not to show it, and their own working relationships may go awry as a result or they may fall victim to emotional burn-out. Because of this, high-stress paediatric areas often have child mental health professionals coming in to consult. They may become involved in staff discussion groups, as well as giving advice on how to deal with specific child problems.

If you would like to have an opportunity to discuss your child's or family's emotional problems with someone a little bit outside the immediate medical system, then you can usually request to see such a counsellor.

Useful organisations

Cystic Fibrosis Research Trust
  Alexandra House
  5 Blyth Road
  Bromley, Kent BR1 3RS
  Tel: 081 464 7211

Provides explanatory leaflets and has a nationwide network of self-help groups.

Friedreich's Ataxia Group
  Copse Edge
  Thursley Road
  Elstead
  Godalming
  Surrey GU8 6DJ
  Tel: 0252 702864

Funds research into the cause of the disease and provides a comprehensive welfare service for all members who suffer from Friedreich's, cerebellar and other ataxia diseases. Offers counselling, finance, equipment, holidays, education and employment. Quarterly magazine and local contacts.

Helen House Hospice for Children
  37 Leopold Street
  Oxford OX4 1QT
  Tel: 0865 728251

Gives respite care to children with a life-threatening disease and helps with terminal care.

Leukaemia Care Society
  14 Kingfisher Court
  Venny Bridge
  Pinhoe
  Exeter
  Devon EX4 8JN
  Tel: 0392 64848

Gives information and support.

Nigel Clare Network Trust
  c/o The Alexandra Gordon Agency
  PO Box 44
  Woking
  Surrey GU21 5TE
  Tel: 0483 724907
Self-help group for parents of children with life-limiting diseases.

Tay Sachs and Allied Diseases Association
  c/o Royal Manchester Children's Hospital
  Hospital Road
  Pendlebury
  Manchester M27 1HA
  Tel: 061 794 4696
Supports affected families.

A CHILD'S DEATH

The death of a child is something that is such a rare and tragic event in our society that people do not know how to prepare for it, when that is possible, or how to behave after it has happened. The other children in the family may be affected very much – sometimes even if they are too young to understand at the time, or are even not yet born.

Maurice was the only child of two comparatively elderly parents who was considerably indulged and over-protected and at the age of eight seemed very immature and disruptive at school. The reasons for his over-protection became apparent at the child guidance unit when his parents revealed that before Maurice was born, four older brothers and sisters had died in a fire at home. They had never discussed this much with Maurice because of their own extreme grief and guilt, and wish to spare his feelings. Maurice's own fantasies revealed a preoccupation with fire, and he needed a long period of therapy to improve, while his parents also received counselling.

———————————◆———————————

Victor was referred to the hospital clinic aged five because of his constant difficult, demanding and aggressive behaviour at school. Although there were still many current stresses on his lone parent mother, things had seemed to go wrong from the pregnancy, which had been of twins. The twins had been born premature and both were very weak. The other twin, also a boy, had died. The father and his family hardly visited at all and did not discuss the death of the twin. The mother's family considered her to be a strong person who would be getting help from the father's side, and so were also not very supportive.

Victor's mother went home with him alone from the hospital to face the clothes and equipment that had been bought for twins. Somehow her emotional attachment to this baby that survived became a very mixed one, so that she sometimes felt so desperate that she just left him suddenly with his father's family. Victor was understandably quite insecure as a result.

When one twin dies, emotions can become quite confused as there is no time to mourn the baby who has died, and the baby who is still alive needs celebration, attention and love.

Deaths of children can be very sudden – as with a traffic accident or even a murder, and such a meaningless and terrible event can cause severe emotional disturbance to the rest of the family even quite a time after the original event.

Lester was referred at 14 to the child guidance unit because his increasingly bad behaviour at school was making it quite probable that he would be expelled. The family was already known to the clinic because an older brother had similiar problems at the same age. The year before, at the age of 16, he had been stabbed to death during an argument in the street. It was not surprising that his mother was now very fearful that yet another son might 'go the same way'.

Other children die after a prolonged period of serious illness. This may not be easier to prepare for, unless there has been a specific turning point when doctors, nurses and parents have together realised and discussed that the end is inevitable, and that measures should now be directed to the child's comfort and happiness rather than to painful and increasingly futile interventions. Intensive care baby units now often allow and encourage parents to hold their babies in their arms when nothing more can be done and share their expression of feelings.

It is best to tell even a two-year-old brother or sister what has happened as they usually know that mummy went into hospital to have a baby and cannot understand if the baby does not appear.

The hospice movement has done a lot to improve the last days of adults dying from cancer, and their philosophy is also becoming available for children. A particular centre for this is:

St Christopher's Hospice
51 Lawrie Park Road
Sydenham
London SE26 6DZ
Tel: 081 778 9252

Some parents want their children to die at home and often
nursing and medical help can be provided so that this is
possible. Brothers and sisters can then take part in the care
of the ill child and this may be an important and
comforting memory for them later on.

Useful organisations

Compassionate Friends
    6 Denmark Street
    Bristol BS1 5DQ
    Tel: 0272 292778
A group of bereaved parents who offer help and understanding to other bereaved parents.

Cruse (Bereavement Care)
    126 Sheen Road
    Richmond
    Surrey TW9 1UR
    Tel: 081 940 4818
Provides bereavement counselling and advice.

Stillbirth and Neonatal Death Society (SANDS)
    28 Portland Place
    London W1N 4DE
    Tel: 071 436 5881
Supports parents who have suffered a stillbirth, late
pregnancy loss or whose baby dies before reaching a
month in age through local self-help groups or individual
befriending.

7

PROBLEMS AT SCHOOL

Many children have some temporary problems at school, perhaps of settling in at infant or secondary stage, or not seeming to progress at all with one particular teacher, or hating particular subjects – whether geography, French or physical education. Usually this sort of problem resolves either just in the course of time or with a bit of help from parents and teachers getting together. For some children, however, difficulties just seem to get worse and outside help of some kind may be necessary.

This chapter looks at some of the kinds of problems that may arise and the type of help available within the education system.

DISRUPTIVE BEHAVIOUR

The kind of bad behaviour that occurs at school is often called 'disruptive behaviour' and parents should always inquire exactly what this means. Often the child seems to be concentrating poorly on what he or she is supposed to be doing and is not only easily distracted by others but gets up and walks around, chatting to and annoying other children.

This can escalate to constant disobedience, cheek to

and defiance of the teacher and even to throwing chairs and actual aggression in the classroom. Temper tantrums in the classroom and defying the authority of the teacher are things teachers understandably do not like as they directly interfere with the orderly education of the whole class.

Your child's misbehaviour, however, is an end-point of a complicated set of circumstances involving the child himself or herself, the other children, the teacher and other staff and even your own relationship with the school and attitudes towards education and authority.

What factors *within the child* might lead to disruptiveness? Suppose your son is not particularly good at reading but is a good mimic, indeed quite a comedian; he finds this gains attention and approval from the other children, which may even be increased by punishment from the teacher.

Another child might be sensitive and prone to temper tantrums; other children quickly find out how to wind him up then step back swiftly leaving him to carry the can when the teacher decides that enough is enough.

What factors *at school* may contribute to this? Children's behaviour is usually better when they are in a clearly structured and well-supervised situation so it is not surprising that complaints about fighting and aggressiveness at playtime and lunchtime are quite common. If a class also has a repeated series of inexperienced teachers, an already vulnerable child will be the one affected.

A challenge to the authority of the school has to be taken seriously by the school, even if you as parents feel that as far as your own child is concerned the school has over-reacted or for the sake of discipline has dealt too strictly with your child. Schools have a number of options open to them – although corporal punishment is no longer one of them. First the class teacher may use the type of penalties available – telling off, keeping in, putting 'on report', giving lines or extra work. Calling in a more senior teacher or sending the child to the head will be used for more serious disciplinary offences. If serious misbehaviour continues then short suspensions from school may be given and these may culminate in expulsion or permanent exclusion.

If the school thinks there may be more to the problem than simply defiance then other resources may be called in. For instance some schools have teachers who are trained in counselling or have specific pastoral responsibilities. Some heads may decide to bring in the education welfare officer or may ask the school's educational psychologist or school doctor for advice. It may be suggested that a change of school would help, or even attendance at a special school. Obviously, the earlier parents are brought into a process of constructive discussion about what to do, the better the outcome is likely to be.

Terry was eight, red-headed, the brighter one of non-identical twins and very lively and tall for his age. Because of his height, his protectiveness towards his twin, self-reliance and a confident even cheeky way with adults he was often thought to be older than he really was. At school he began to get into more and more trouble for cheekiness and disobedience and for getting into fights with other children. Terry's parents were devoted to their children, giving them a lot materially, but also lots of time and attention. They were mystified as to why Terry should be the source of so much trouble at school and felt he must be being picked on as they could not believe he was the only naughty boy there. However, they did admit that he could be a handful, and was particularly rude and difficult with his mother, though better behaved with his father.

Terry's parents did what they could, including looking at dietary problems at the school's suggestions and constantly going to the school to take Terry out when there was an episode of disturbance, which became a considerable source of stress to the family. Terry did quite well when in a class with an experienced teacher, but was difficult when his usual teacher was away sick. He was suspended several times and expulsion was threatened. The school was reluctant to move him to a different class from his twin because it was not their policy to separate twins.

Eventually both Terry's parents decided that a change of school had to be tried, to give him a chance in another situation where they felt he would not be instantly labelled as a troublemaker. At the same time they had, with the help of the child guidance clinic, successfully modified their approach to handling Terry at home, being firmer rather than getting into long debates about who had started it, what was on his mind and so forth.

◆

Todd, aged 11, was referred to the child psychiatrist by a paediatrician. He had recently been found to have a mild form of epilepsy which was responding well to medication. However, he had been expelled from his primary school for disruptive behaviour and there seemed to be no signs of him gaining another place at a school, although he had been provided with an individual tutor (sometimes known as a home tutor) for a few hours a week.

Todd was seen with his family which consisted of his mother and father and an older sister. Todd was overweight and strikingly immature. It emerged that he could also be a terrible pest at home – mainly rowing with his sister – and the parents seemed very stressed by this. He seemed to take little responsibility – for instance he did not even dress himself. And on the educational side he could not read except for little words such as 'and' or 'is'.

It turned out that before Todd was born there had been another son who had been mentally handicapped and had died at the age of two. In addition, when Todd was three he had been sexually abused by an older boy on the estate. These factors seemed to have led to understandable protectiveness and indulgence from his parents – but unfortunately to the point where Todd's appropriate development was becoming impaired.

Todd was assessed by the clinical psychologist at the clinic and surprisingly his intelligence was average and he did not have any of the specific features of dyslexia. It appeared he had learned not to learn and the extent of his under-achievement had not been recognised by his school. The school psychologist was asked to help, and the 'Full Assessment Procedure' for special education started (see page 167), while family treatment continued at the clinic.

◆

Janine, aged 14, was referred to the child guidance unit by her school. She was the kind of girl who always pushed authority to its limits – for instance if the wearing of small sleeper earrings was allowed, she would wear large hoops. If make-up was forbidden she would have on lipstick and mascara. She often seemed to be behind disturbances in the classroom and her attitude annoyed many of the teachers.

Janine's parents were angry with Janine for the trouble she was causing, angry with the school for apparently picking on Janine and angry at 'having' to come to the clinic. They also wondered if the fact that Janine's mother was black and her father white was contributing to the difficulties, as the church school where Janine attended did not usually have many black pupils. It was true that Janine was not a disturbed girl and there were none of the distressing family circumstances which characterise so many of the referrals to the clinic.

Janine's parents considered the options: should they change her school, increase their disapproval and punishment if she misbehaved or say it was up to Janine? They felt they had already done what they could and the misdemeanours complained of often seemed trivial.

The clinic was able to offer a mediating role once the parents had decided to keep Janine at the same school and arranged a joint meeting. Janine was also seen regularly by herself at the clinic to help her consider her own interest in achieving qualifications at school.

What parents can do

It is a nasty shock for parents when they are asked to go to the school to discuss their child's misbehaviour. It reminds them of their own school days when they felt small and fearful of the authority of the head, and it becomes very difficult to have an adult-to-adult conversation on equal terms. That is probably why you may feel an urge either to be very quiet, apologetic and agree to any suggestion or alternatively to become angry with the school and defensive about your child. Sometimes the behaviour complained of seems completely trivial and something that you feel the school should have coped with on their own; sometimes it seems as if your child is being picked on for not fitting in somehow.

It's not easy, but try to keep in your mind that you know your child best – both his or her strengths and weaknesses, so the school is going to need your expertise if in any difficulty with your child. First of all try to establish the details – where, when, how often, what preceded the misbehaviour, what happened next and so forth, but do this in a spirit of joint inquiry. It may emerge that there are some simple measures that could be tried by the school such as ensuring the oversight of an experienced teacher or requesting extra reading help for your child.

Ask how the school thinks you can help – for example you might offer to come in once a week to discuss progress. Go for an approach that involves as many positives as possible, rather than punishment, for instance a report card coming home daily which notes achievements as well as misdeeds.

It helps if both parents can visit the school together, even if otherwise they are separated. If you cannot bring your partner then, especially if it looks as if expulsion is a possibility, bring another relative or friend or a community worker. Sometimes an educational welfare officer can be helpful, or if your family is already seeing someone from a child guidance or child psychiatry clinic then they may be usefully involved.

Repeated suspensions are rarely a successful method of improving behaviour, so if this point is reached you should ask what other resources for help the school has access to, and also consider moving your child to another school. The child may respond better in a different setting.

As far as expulsion procedures are concerned, normally parents may attend a hearing at which the governors are present and may bring a friend or representative. If the child is suspended or expelled, he or she is entitled to education but sometimes there are long delays before alternatives are offered – and these may be far from satisfactory.

Of course, it is far better to start to work in alliance with the school as early as possible to avoid the occasion for expulsion. If you acknowledge that your child has faults, explain any difficulties you have at home that may be contributing and show that you are willing to do what you can, then teachers will also feel encouraged to try again. The main advice to parents is to keep calm over your child's difficulties, and work it out with the school.

TRUANCY

If your child is ill at home, obviously you know that your child is not attending school and why. Some children, however, leave home in the morning as if to go to school, but in fact go off to the park or shopping centre with friends – in other words they play truant. A variant of this is bunking off for some or many lessons, often after registration.

Unaccounted for absence from school is rare in primary schools, which are near to home and have a relatively small community of staff and pupils. Truancy increases throughout the secondary school years with attendance rates of less than 75 per cent being common in the last two years of compulsory education.

It can take some time for parents to become aware of what is happening. Schools always check attendance, but catching up with only partial or intermittent bunking off is quite difficult. And although schools will notify parents if there is unexplained non-attendance, children have been known to pay close attention to the post and destroy the evidence! Schools will also draw persistent non-attendance to the attention of the education welfare service who are likely to visit the home to see what is happening.

If you are very unlucky, the first you may know of your child's truancy is a call from the police about some trouble such as shop-lifting or glue-sniffing.

Derek, aged 14, did not go to school very much at all. He was not very academically successful, but had never received any special help. As he was not there on the days that the final two years' options were being chosen it looked as if he would be assigned to courses which held no interest for him. For a while, he had been offered a place at a support unit within the school; he had enjoyed this more because of the simplified curriculum and the close supervision by a small staff. However, this term other children had a higher priority for the unit, and the particular teacher that Derek had learned to trust had left.

Unfortunately, this school had a very high truancy rate so once again Derek's needs did not seem particularly outstanding. Derek's parents went to their GP for advice and were referred on to the child guidance clinic. There they discussed how they had many difficulties themselves, and were not particularly ambitious for Derek. They were not hostile to education and knew that he could be putting himself at risk of delinquency if he was just allowed to roam with friends or older boys. However, they had little idea of what they could do. The clinic staff were able to help the family, school and education welfare service get together to sort out a more acceptable and attractive educational programme for Derek, and to ensure that a continued personal interest was taken in his good attendance and progress.

Robin, aged 13, was brought to the clinic by his parents at the request of the education welfare service. He was the eldest of two children and had been playing truant from school frequently. He had been twice picked up by the police in the city centre during school hours and was suspected of shop-lifting, though he denied it. Robin's mother was quite distraught, but his father was not as concerned – he felt that school had not done him much good, and yet he had done reasonably well in life.

Robin was an articulate and cheerful boy, defiant of authority. He said school was 'boring and useless', and gave many instances of how he was unjustly 'picked on' for minor details such as having the wrong shoes, refusing to wear a tie and so forth. He even knew what the solution was; he wanted to go to a unit like some of his older friends, where the kids were allowed to wear what they liked and the discipline seemed to be less strict.

What parents can do

It can be seen that truancy is a difficult problem to tackle alone. If you are fortunate enough to be informed at an early stage by the school then you should take this issue very seriously with your child and also ensure that the school informs you every time that the child is not present. Some schools are not very good at that, unlike some schools in the United States whose computers can ring up parents with information about truants.

Try to talk calmly to your son or daughter to discover what it is that they dislike about school. Discuss ways of putting those things right, and also talk through how they might avoid pressure from friends who are urging them to bunk off.

Parents need to become allies with the school but they

may develop a feeling that the school is quite happy not to
see some of the 14- to 16-year-olds who are not concentrating on exams and are generally disaffected. If that
happens to be the case, ask if some other kind of provision
such as a support unit or other small unit in or near the
school is available. These are quite successful with truants
who may find the approach more individualistic and
acceptable.

But the best possible way of overcoming the problem is
for the parent to work very closely with the school. It is
essential the problem is not ignored; increasing truancy
can lead to severe delinquency, like drug-taking and
prostitution.

BULLYING

Children rarely speak to adults about being bullied,
perhaps because of feeling ashamed or because they have
not found it to be of any help in the past. Yet bullying is
very common in schools and a source of much unhappiness for the victims. It may take various forms – both
physical and verbal – but is often persistent and threatening. Sometimes the object is to get the victim to give up
possessions or money; and this kind of extortion is widespread and may continue for months without any adults
being aware of what is happening.

Unpleasant teasing is also common and distressing.
Children these days do not merely taunt their traditional
butts: the odd-looking, the red-headed, the wearers of
glasses and the plump. They find the sensitive points of
many with insults and name-calling about skin colour and
racial group, about imagined sexual inclination or behaviour. A particular favourite is insulting a child's
mother.

It's very difficult to get children to admit this sort of thing. Unless you ask they will not tell you. Perhaps their father has just left and the child is more sensitive than usual at having aspersions cast on his mother. Sometimes what looks like inexplicable tantrums or anxieties are actually a reaction to this teasing.

Peter was referred to the child guidance clinic by his school's educational psychologist.

Aged 12, Peter came to Britain with his parents and older brother and sister three years ago after a happy life in Zimbabwe. He still missed that country, its warmth, the people and his school very much.

A pale, anxious boy, he was very unhappy at his British school – so much so that he spent all his time in the school library. He said this was due to bullying especially by one boy. He was taken to school by his father, otherwise he would simply not have made it because of bullying on the bus.

His unhappiness and anxiety soon spread through his entire life and he didn't enjoy anything at home and had no friends; the one he did have moved away from the area. He felt British children were rougher than his classmates in Zimbabwe. He found it impossible to fight, either physically or verbally, and when he was angry he went off and punched his pillow. Sometimes he felt so bad he punched his tummy. He found it hard to sleep because of worrying at night about school.

Peter was close to his mother and felt that she also missed Zimbabwe as she shouted at him since leaving. He couldn't tell what his father felt. He quarrelled a lot with his older sister, but she always won. He felt he was the baby and must always lose.

When the therapist was talking to the family, they all spoke about 'London children' as if these were a race apart with whom it was difficult to communicate. The father thought Peter was visibly withdrawn at home, didn't seem to have much fun and was often irritable, especially with his sister. And his mother agreed that Peter was easily upset. Both parents had strong religious convictions which forbade retaliation against aggression, and indeed any expression of anger was strongly disapproved of within the family.

Fortunately, a few family sessions exploring these sorts of issues helped the family to think through the losses and disappointments they had all experienced on coming to Britain and to work out together how best to help Peter. After looking at a number of options, his parents arranged for him to go to a smaller and less demanding school where he was much happier.

◆

Sally, aged 14, was referred to the child guidance clinic by an educational welfare officer. Over the last year, especially the last term, Sally had become the focus of teasing, threats and fights at school, mostly from a group of about four girls. This escalated into name calling and then into phone calls to Sally – sometimes as many as 20 or 30 a night. It was so bad that the family had been driven to changing their phone number. But then threatening letters were received.

Sally's parents informed the police but finally decided not to pursue this line for fear of causing further trouble locally. The head had told the family he would expel the other girls, but did not do so even when the threats and harassment continued. Instead he tried to mediate between the parties but this failed and Sally ran out of the school and refused to return.

The educational welfare officer visited and was

pleasant but threatened possible court proceedings. As the family was unable to afford private education they were beginning to consider educating their daughter at home.

Sally's mother was very uncertain about her daughter seeing a psychiatrist, believing it should be the offenders who were seen. She was very tense, guarded and close to tears. The father was anti-psychiatry. The whole affair had caused marital problems.

With some reluctance the family revealed that Sally had recently twice cut her wrists under the pressure. She had also been neglecting herself, not bathing as much and crying. She never went out by herself.

Fortunately, it was possible to reduce the confrontation with the education system, the threat of court proceedings was dropped and Sally was offered the opportunity of some individual tuition, to which she responded well. However, she remained upset at the very thought of going to another school or even college.

What parents can do

If you suspect that your child is being bullied, ask him or her to tell you about it and what they do when it happens. You may be able to give helpful advice yourself, especially about whether and when it is all right to hit back or to tell a teacher. You may find, by talking with other children and parents, that there is a particular child or group of children who are always involved in the bullying, and if so, it would be sensible to get in touch with the school.

Some schools have developed clear policies on how to react to bullying and so can deal with matters in a much more capable way that is seen by everyone as being fair. If your child's school does not seem to be clear about how to handle bullying, then it is worthwhile raising the issue hrough the Parent Teachers' Association or by contacting one of the school governors. An ideal approach would be one that encouraged co-operative behaviour from all the children while also making the rules of acceptable behaviour clear.

If your own child has been badly affected by bullying, or even perhaps seems to provoke bullying from many children, then psychological help may be needed.

POOR EDUCATIONAL PROGRESS

Children may fall behind the educational achievements of others at school for a variety of reasons:

Some may have a general learning delay, sometimes but not always evident from a young age.

Some may have more specific difficulties of hearing, language development, attention or physical skill.

Some may have missed crucial stages of school through illness or family moves.

Some may have experienced such stress, either recently or over a long period, that anxiety is making it difficult for them to learn.

Commonly it is not always that easy at first to tell what sort of problem is affecting the child in question. Parents will know, however, if there were signs of developmental delay under five, or if there were major life stresses such as a serious hospital operation or a family breakdown. As parents you will also know whether your child was functioning well previously, or if the problems have only started recently. It is often parents, in fact, who draw the issue to the attention of the school especially if the lag is in important basic skills such as reading and writing.

Vanessa, aged seven, was referred to the child guidance unit because during the previous term in the infants she was spiteful to other children, rude to the teacher and not learning properly. At the same time she had been readily upset and difficult at home. However, over the long summer holiday there had been no problems at home. She had settled down better in school with a new teacher so far this term. Vanessa's mother wondered if she might be dyslexic or perhaps a bit deaf – she did have frequent earaches and other members of the family had hearing problems. At the family interview no obvious major past or current stresses emerged; if anything it seemed that Vanessa was upset by school, rather than that another emotional disturbance was causing a learning failure.

Further assessment was recommended, especially of Vanessa's hearing and her general ability. A meeting was arranged at school with the educational psychologist, education social worker and teachers, to which her parents were invited. It turned out that Vanessa's hearing was normal but that she did have a limited educational ability which would need special help. This made a lot of sense to the parents who had also tried themselves to coach Vanessa, but without success.

For the following year Vanessa received extra help within the school, but although useful this did not prove to be sufficient. The Full Assessment procedure was started and eventually Vanessa was placed in a special day school for children with moderate learning difficulties, where she settled in very well.

———————— ◆ ————————

Colin, aged five, was referred to the clinic because of problems of rudeness and wetting. His mother was also concerned that he was failing to learn to read and to take things in in general. In his personality Colin was a quiet and sensitive boy who tended to be a bit of a loner at school. He had started walking at 18 months but had not spoken clearly until about three-and-a-half. However, at a recent developmental check-up his mother had been surprised to hear that he had performed one test at a six-and-a-half-year-old level.

The family had been through a series of crises in the previous year, including separation from the father of the two children after violent rows and the mother breaking away completely from her own family when she discovered that her father had been sexually abusing her small daughter (Colin's younger sister).

Colin was a responsive little boy who drew well for his age although his speech was unclear. He said that he would like to be like He-man on TV because he beats up nasty people. The birds in his picture had sad faces and his mother commented that he always drew sad faces, although it had not occurred to her before that he might be sad.

The psychiatrist wondered if Colin himself had been sexually abused and asked the mother to consider this possibility. She later asked Colin and found that this was probably the case. Social services were then involved, with the mother's agreement, but, as is often the case unfortunately, further investigations with such young children were not conclusive enough for any legal action to be taken against the abuser. Nevertheless, the mother was supported by a social worker from the clinic in beginning to think through her own complex emotions at the same time as safeguarding the children. Sessions of regular individual child psychotherapy were arranged for Colin.

———————◆———————

Craig was 10 when he was referred to the child guidance unit. He was brought by his father, who was
clearly very worried about his son. Craig still could not
recognise words unless there was a picture to help him.
Craig's father said that the problem was long-standing
and that he had felt at first that the professionals were
making light of it. However, the current school
accepted that Craig had a specific learning difficulty
and had arranged for extra help.

In addition the family had been severely upset the
previous year because the mother had fairly suddenly
left the country to live with a man she had met while
they were holidaying abroad. It was evident that
Craig's father still felt very sad when thinking about
this; Craig by contrast was fidgety and reluctant to talk
about his mother at all.

More detailed psychological assessment of Craig's
abilities and achievements was arranged and Craig was
offered regular sessions with the clinic's specialist
teacher, while his father was seen by a psychiatric social
worker. Progress was very slow, but the family was
being supported emotionally to help Craig make the
best educational progress possible.

What parents can do

If your child seems to be making poor educational
progress then the first thing to do is talk this over with his
or her class teacher. Preferably do not leave this until a
special open evening or you may find that explanations are
being asked of you, or the teacher may not even have
considered that there was a problem and so has not had
time to think about it.

Think yourself about whether there were earlier signs of
developmental delay, whether it seems as if there is a

special problem with reading, or whether something might have upset your child at school or at home.

There may be quite simple things that the school and parents can co-operate on to re-establish the child's learning progress. Or there may be a need for further specialist assessment by a teacher or educational psychologist, or perhaps at the local child guidance unit. If you think your child needs help, then do persist; even if your boy or girl is not going to be an academic high-flier you will still want him or her to have the best chances possible, and you are entitled to ask the education authority for an assessment to see if there are 'special educational needs'.

As in the cases above, there can be quite a complex mixture of difficulties sometimes. Nevertheless, even when there are a lot of emotional problems and therapy of some sort at a child guidance unit is offered, the child is also likely to need specific extra educational help.

WHEN THE SCHOOL IS THE PROBLEM

Schools under stress

Schools as institutions can also be under stress just as much as a family: if there are a lot of legislative changes, political interventions, budgetary problems, union disputes or difficulties in recruiting then this can add up to a very stressed school with less to give to the children. Many schools have been undergoing all of these experiences in recent years, with resultant loss of morale and increased staff sickness and turnover.

Parents, however, may have very little idea of what is happening in the staffroom, but may become aware that their child is getting into more trouble or becoming more anxious or not learning much any more. If you speak to other parents and check out the situation you may find out that it is not just your child who is reacting badly.

Parents can go to the head teacher and to the governors to tell them of their concerns. It may be that a joint approach to the local education authority can provide some remedy if, for instance, resources are really the problem. Or there may be some other way in which the parents and the local community can help. But to put right a school that has gone badly wrong can take months, if not years, and is the responsibility of the local education authority. You do need to consider how to safeguard your own child while this is going on. Is it worth changing schools for instance, or is the company of friends and the presence of one or two trusted teachers enough support?

Sexual molestation at school

The fact that a teacher may have had inappropriate physical contact with a child is hardly something that would occur to most parents worried about their child's unhappiness at school. But again, if several parents become worried that something is happening to their child, and on comparing notes find a similar situation, it must be taken very seriously. The parents should go to the head of the school with another person – a friend or another parent, especially one whose child is also involved.

If a parent, or parents, are agreed that there are serious grounds for concern and the head is uncertain or reluctant to take any steps, the parents should write to the Director of the local education department whose name and address can be found from the town hall. They should also consider contacting the police. Once such a complaint or allegation is in writing, then there will have to be a formal investigation. Of course, you will have to bear in mind that your child may be questioned and that this itself may

e stressful, though children are sometimes more matter-
f-fact about these things than adults.

Parents should not underestimate the possibility of
exual abuse within a school – especially if the child has a
isability of some kind or is at a boarding school. Some
chool systems go very wrong for many years and children
r even staff are not believed.

SOURCES OF HELP IN SCHOOLS

The school health service

Generally schools have regular visits from a school doctor
nd a school nurse who are not just there to look for nits
nd do eye-tests, but to play an important part in ensuring
hat children's health needs are looked after so that they
an benefit from their education.

They can investigate if there are health difficulties lying
ehind any failure to progress, and can also explain
iedical conditions such as asthma, eczema or epilepsy to
eachers. Sometimes children or parents like to discuss first
ith the school doctor or nurse a number of private
orries, and they can then be referred on if appropriate.

A medical examination and report is an essential part
f the Full Assessment for special education needs pro-
edure.

The education welfare service

ine of the major roles of the education welfare service (or
ducation social work service, as it is sometimes called) is
provide help with truancy. Education social workers
ay be attached to a specific group of schools or have
sponsibility for a specific local patch. Schools usually
otify instances of persistent unaccounted for absence to

their education social workers who will follow it up with home visits. The ESWs will then do all they can to find out what the problem is by talking to the parents, making friends with the child and mediating at school. They can also help with general welfare issues such as benefits, housing and holidays, as well as supporting and guiding parents through the special education procedures. As social workers they also have a responsibility within schools for liaison with social services about children who may be 'at risk'.

If truancy persists the education welfare service may take legal action. A child can no longer be taken into care solely for non-attendance, but parents and child may have to go to court and the child may become subject to an Education Supervision Order. This might mean an education social worker working to improve the attendance by visiting the child at home, closely supervising attendance and providing any other necessary help and advice.

Contacting the education welfare service is one way of obtaining help for your child. You can be referred by the school, contact the service direct or be referred by another professional like a teacher or a social worker.

The education welfare service is run by the local authority, either as part of the education or the social services department. You can find the address and telephone number in the phone book or via the town hall, local library or Citizens' Advice Bureau.

Education psychologists

If the problem with the child appears, from the parents' point of view, to be not just a behaviour problem but also one in which the child is behind academically, then they are entitled to ask for more assessment and help and an educational psychologist might be asked to assess the child.

Whether the problems are behavioural, academic or both, the educational psychologist may observe the child in the classroom to see how he or she approaches their work. The child may also be interviewed alone or with the parents, and tested for ability and attainment. After consulting with the parents, the psychologist may advise the teacher and suggest a change of curriculum or of approach, or recommend some special help inside or outside the school.

Special educational provision

If parents feel their child has special education needs and want something extra from the educational system they have a right to make a request directly to the local educational authority for their child to undergo a Full Assessment Procedure. Alternatively, the school itself or the educational psychologist may initiate this – with the agreement of the parents. The end result, often after considerable – even prolonged – assessment should be a 'statement' of the child's special education needs and how the authority proposes to meet them. It does not necessarily mean that the child will be offered special school placement; it may be possible to provide support within the school.

Results of recent educational changes such as the national curriculum, local management of schools and standardised assessment may work to the disadvantage of difficult or educationally needy children as they may be seen as 'expensive' and lowering a school's results average.

Various types of special educational help may be available.

Extra help within school

Children with a variety of minor difficulties leading to lack of progress may be helped by extra teaching help within the school. This may be individual or on a small group basis. Sometimes a general assistant is provided when it is felt that an extra adult would enable the class teacher to deal with, say, a disabled or very difficult child. Some help is often available without a Full Assessment, but if substantial help will be needed over a prolonged period then a Full Assessment 'statement' is usually necessary.

Part-time off-site

Children may be sent to a smaller class for part of the week, sometimes a special tutorial class, which may be held at the school or what is called 'off-site' – in a room or hall away from the school.

Full-time off-site

It is sometimes suggested that older children whose behaviour is difficult attend a support unit either at, or near, the school.

Parents need to look at this suggestion very carefully. What does the curriculum there offer? What is the record of success? Do they succeed in getting the child back into the ordinary mainstream school and, if so, on what time scale? Do they concentrate as much on the child's learning difficulties as their behaviour? What is their attendance rate?

Parents should inquire very closely about these matters before agreeing as they are bound to be worried about the possible effects on the child of taking exams in this system, any possible stigma the child might feel at being transferred and any effects on the child at being associated with even more disturbed children, which may make them worse.

However, many of these units are successful and

popular with previously disaffected pupils as the staff can concentrate more on the individual needs of children within a small group. This improves the children's self-esteem as well as getting them more attuned to learning again.

Special schools

Various types of school come under this heading and parents must look very closely at which provision they think will suit their particular child. Some authorities have been trying to provide more integrated provision since the 1981 Education Act, but there are often special schools for children with moderate or severe learning difficulties, for emotionally and behaviourally disturbed children, for delicate children and for autistic children as well as those for more obvious physical, sight and hearing handicaps.

The advantages of segregated special education may be that the child can receive specialist attention in a smaller and less rejecting group, where he or she may feel less different. Some children really thrive in such a placement, but a lot depends on the actual school and the individual child. The disadvantages may be removal from the 'normal' peer group, leading to a feeling of stigmatisation, and loss of access to the challenge and range of the full curriculum.

Another option that parents may have to consider is special boarding education. This can be very useful sometimes, especially if the child is so provocative that family as well as school relationships are near breaking point, or if family stress is so high that a child simply cannot concentrate.

Useful organisations

Advisory Centre For Education
   18 Aberdeen Studios
   22–24 Highbury Grove
   London N5 2EA
   Tel: 071 354 8321

National education watchdog body which presses for a fairer and more responsive education system. Gives free advice and support to parents of children in state schools.

Children's Legal Centre
   20 Compton Terrace
   London N1 2UN
   Tel: 071 359 6251

Provides advice and information on all legal matters relating to children and young people.

8

THE NON-TRADITIONAL FAMILY

The average family of two parents, two children and a dog, certainly still exists and attracts a lot of advice. But these days there are many other kinds of household in which children are brought up. How can the parents or responsible adults find the help they may need if their children are having emotional difficulties? What particular problems may they face, or find especially hard to cope with?

The number of non-traditional families is growing. Now almost 30 per cent of children are born to mothers who are not married to the father and there are over one million lone parent families in the United Kingdom. So many children spend some part of their childhood being looked after by one parent alone; this may be because the mother has been alone from the outset, or because of divorce, separation or death.

Although our culture expects the mother to be the main carer for children this is not always the case; the father may be the lone parent and grandparents also often take over as carers, especially if the parents are very young. Some children, whose original ('birth') parents cannot look after them well enough, may be taken into the care of the local authority and subsequently adopted or fostered.

And so foster and adoptive parents also have particular challenges to face.

Now that one marriage in three breaks up the numbers of step-children are growing, along with the complications this set of relationships brings. It is not unusual for there to be two sets of children from both partners' previous marriages, then a child or children from the current marriage. This can naturally create problems.

Finally, although in a minority, there are children who are being brought up by declared or undeclared gay or lesbian couples.

THE LONE MOTHER

In the last 20 years it has become much more common for a parent (usually the mother) to bring up a child alone. Lone parent families now make up 17 per cent of all families in Britain.

This situation may be deliberately planned. Some young women become pregnant more or less accidentally and decide to be single mothers if the father is not particularly interested or supportive. A significant number of more mature women also make a conscious decision to take this path.

However, it is very difficult to take sole responsibility for a child, and there are many stresses on such a parent from the purely economic, through the many practical difficulties of juggling with child-minding and employment, to social isolation and exhaustion. Obviously these are stresses that affect the child too. And although the small family of mother alone with a single child is not uncommon these days, by the time the child is four-years-old he or she will begin to pick up the idea that 'everyone else has a mummy and daddy – where is my daddy?' In fact the fathers are rarely completely out of the picture but may, from the mother's and child's point of view, be un-reliable and a cause of continuing conflict.

Bill, for instance, was three. His mother brought him to the clinic because he was suffering from nightmares. The previous year she had made an attempt to renew her relationship with Bill's father. Bill had made her feel 'gutted' when at a Christmas family occasion he had asked publicly 'Who is that man, Mummy?' Then the little boy had got to know his father and they got on very well in each other's company, but the parents' relationship broke down again. His mother tried to arrange for Bill to stay for weekends with his father, but this only happened on a few occasions as the father felt his freedom was being restricted too much.

◆

Joseph was brought at the age of four to the clinic by his mother because she thought he was hyperactive, and that the occasional contacts that he had with his father and his father's family were upsetting him. She also saw in him the very worst personality character-istics that had led her not to make a permanent rela-tionship with his father.

The children's views in such a situation can often only be guessed at. But often they try to maintain an idealised view of the missing father, and boys especially may become quite aggressive and angry with their mothers.

As a lone parent you have to be both father and mother, and so have to be the one who sets the limits, as well as the one who loves and comforts. As you may also be working full-time and so very busy, sometimes your child may get too little of either warmth or control.

Boys in a situation like this seem particularly likely to come off badly when there are no other supports such as relatives, friends, a new step-father or good child-care arrangements.

> Dennis, for instance, was referred by his school at the age of eight because he seemed rather miserable but also aggressive and consequently had few friends. It turned out that he was the only child of a single mother who had only recently left her own parents' home as she had managed to acquire her own flat. However, this meant for Dennis that he often had to be at home all alone, as his mother was working full-time, and he missed the company and care of the wider family.
>
> Although the mother often could not come to the clinic, fortunately when the school understood more of the circumstances they began to work with her to improve things – encouraging Dennis to learn the French horn and take part in after-school activities. A goldfish was bought as a pet for Dennis, and he and his mother became appreciably happier and more relaxed.

What can you as a lone mother do to help prevent your child having emotional problems? First, if there is a father around who has some interest then it helps the child to maintain this relationship – even if the adults do not agree with each other over many things, or the child seems to be 'upset' by visits. Families do find successful methods to get round this – a good way is to use a more neutral person such as the father's mother, who may be able to offer a visiting base where the child and father can meet. The new Children Act encourages this kind of joint parental responsibility as being in the child's best interest, and hopefully statutory and voluntary agencies will develop more facilities for mediation and access facilities.

If contact with their real father is an impossibility, nevertheless it is still very important especially for boys to have positive, continuing relationships with men whom they can admire and respect. Sometimes lone mothers understandably spend a lot of time in each other's company for support – but this may encourage an attitude that all men are unreliable or aggressive, and produce a generation of boys who think exactly that.

So who would you like your son to respect, imitate and be able to trust? A grandfather may be only too willing to take his grandson fishing but may need to be asked to take a special interest. Or an uncle might be persuaded to go to the school's open evening with you. Even if you are not generally a practising Christian, think about having a named god father or two for your son. Or join a social, family group activity where fathers also take part – perhaps a church or a community education centre. Activities for boys such as sports clubs or scouts can also be useful and relieve the pressure on you to take the sole responsibility for your son – which may lead either to an over-close relationship or considerable tension.

Make sure too that you have some leisure time to call your own if at all possible, so that each generation can take part in the natural interests of their own age-group.

Professional support really cannot provide satisfactory alternatives to friends and family relationships, though sometimes advice or counselling may be helpful for support and guidance if you as the parent feel over-whelmed by difficulties.

Many women now become lone parents after separation or divorce and a smaller number are left alone through widowhood. If you are in this situation, you are more likely to have more than one child, thus avoiding some of the 'hot-house' effects described above, but are likely to go through a period of severe stress. Some similar issues arise: how can you be both the firm person and the comforter? How can you give sufficient attention to the children if you are exhausted by work and financial worries? If you are under stress it can be really too much of an effort to do anything but scream ineffectively when the children get out of hand (which they will).

Child guidance staff quite often see families in which the level of exhaustion and depression of the lone mother seems to match the excessive noise and out-of-control behaviour of the children in what is clearly a vicious circle.

An extreme example is provided by Francine, who was a very tall seven-year-old when she came to the hospital department with her family. The problem was that she was boisterous and disobedient at school, demanding constant attention and trying to extend the limits of any boundaries set. She was the youngest of five children. Her father had left the family five years before and was seen occasionally but did not provide much financial or emotional support.

Francine was sad her father was not at home. Francine's difficult behaviour tended to drive her mother to ask for the father's help, but she felt she only received criticism and blame. Francine's mother spoke very quietly and she had a stammer. It was clear she was not used to exerting authority successfully.

Problems of control are common for lone parents. Some think that children ought to behave well naturally, and that if they don't it is somehow the absent parent's fault – whether because of genetics, a bad example or for other reasons. Sometimes the child picks up something of this and may work out that a good way to see Dad again is to be so bad that he is called in as the authority figure.

Ian was 14 and the younger of two children. The parents had been divorced two years before, with the children staying with their mother but seeing their father regularly. Ian was a very bright boy who had been doing well at school, but had started to refuse to attend. This led to terrible scenes with his mother every morning, and as she was not getting anywhere she began to try to get his father on the phone to deal with it. Needless to say, this was quite ineffective, but in some way suited the emotional position of each parent. The mother could go on pointing out how difficult her son was and how unhelpful his father was. The father could maintain that his wife was unreasonably demanding and also an ineffective parent.

A lone parent may come to the clinic hoping that others can 'make' their child behave and be surprised to find that it is a change in their own attitude and approach which may be necessary.

To take a contrasting example, Mrs Green from the start of the family's contact with the clinic wanted the main support and advice of the staff to be for herself. Although her 12-year-old son Robert was extremely difficult – he was stealing, wetting and lying – she had some insight into why this might be. She and her husband had been through a painful divorce a few years previously, in which her husband sought and gained custody of his daughter only. Subsequently, the girl was given much more materially and emotionally by her father and his parents than Robert, who was only too aware of the contrast.

Mrs Green felt hurt by her daughter's apparent rejection of her, and she also seemed to be the object of Robert's angry feelings. However, on the whole she

managed not to continue a cycle of retaliation with her
ex-husband and used counselling help sensibly to help
cope with her own complex feelings and the challenging behaviour of her son.

THE LONE FATHER

Less often the lone parent is a father. If you are in this
position, you too will have the problems of combining the
roles of father and mother, unless other women step in to
help. You will also discover that child-care and employment are extremely difficult to manage together successfully, and may yourself be receiving undeserved blame or
criticism from the children.

In recent years there has been a rise in the number of
mothers leaving their children when they are quite young,
and this is a very sad and difficult thing to explain to
children. Again, it is not easy to provide appropriately for
the developing needs of a child of the opposite sex – in
this case the daughter – and special arrangements may be
needed.

Professional agencies are also much more used to the
lone mother than the lone father. So, if you are in this
position and would like specialist advice about family
issues, ask around as to where might be the most suitable
source. You might prefer an agency which has experience
of advising fathers – where some of the staff are men and
may even be fathers themselves.

Useful organisations

Families Need Fathers
    BM Families
    London WC1N 3XX
    Tel: 081 886 0970
Helps and advises fathers wanting to remain in contact with their family.

Gingerbread
    35 Wellington Street
    London WC2 7BN
    Tel: 071 240 0953
Helps and supports lone parent families through a national network of self-help groups.

National Council For One Parent Families
    255 Kentish Town Road
    London NW5 2LX
    Tel: 071 267 1361
Provides information.

STEP-PARENTS

Nobody has ever said that family life is easy, though the long-term rewards may be great – and this applies even more to step-families. When does a step-family start being one anyway? When does Mum's regular boyfriend become a step-father?

Technically the answer may be when they marry, but that really reflects the legal relationship between two adults of the opposite sex, not the emotional relationship between each adult and the other spouse's children – who may or may not be living in the same household.

The problem of roles instantly arises. Does each parent/step-parent have an equal right to set rules for the children and discipline them, or responsibility to take them to the dentist or talk to the school? What about the rights and responsibilities of the non-custodial parent (usually the one who does not have the children living permanently with them)?

These sorts of issues may be highlighted, rather than lessened, when along comes the joint product of the new relationship – a baby. Sadly, the older children may then feel rather pushed out as the specialness of their relationship with their 'real' parent is reduced. A vicious cycle can easily occur in step-relationships, with each party feeling that all their best efforts are rejected. A mother living with her children and a new husband may feel forced to take sides – and then someone is bound to feel let down.

> Lester's mother, Mrs White, for instance was rightly concerned when her 10-year-old son had recurrent episodes of pain and vomiting and agreed with the paediatrician's suggestion that this might be connected with family stresses. When she brought Lester to see the child psychiatrist it emerged that she had separated from Lester's father five years previously and had a two-year-old son by her new partner. However, there were continuing rows about how and when Lester's father could visit him, and Mrs White also felt her current partner was treating Lester unfairly. Although she tried to keep the actual quarrels away from the children, nevertheless she also tended, rather inappropriately, to confide in Lester and ask him for advice. In fact, it had got to the point where she was seriously considering leaving with the children.

———◆———

Paul, aged six, was brought to the clinic by his step-mother, Mrs Williams, who found him totally exasperating as he was rude, rejecting and disobedient towards her, and aggressive towards her own slightly older daughter Katrina. Mrs Williams felt angry that she seemed to be expected to do all the caring for and the disciplining of Paul – with no reliable and regular support from his 'real' mother – while Mr Williams seemed very laid back about it all and didn't really see that there was any problem.

Mrs Williams had had an unhappy life herself, including violent relationships and several miscarriages. She felt very strongly attached to Paul, but at the same time she found him almost unbearable to be with to the point that she wanted him in boarding school, or else she threatened to end the marriage.

———————◆———————

Patrick was brought to the hospital clinic by his mother because he seemed unhappy, withdrawn and was not making good progress at school. Patrick's father had died. He had three older brothers and his mother had recently remarried a widower who had three children, not yet grown up and similar in age to Patrick's family. Although all parties were trying hard to make things work, one may imagine that there was suddenly a lot of competition for things, from bedroom space to mother's attention. The rules and standards of the two families were naturally not identical, so many decisions made in the interests of peace seemed to Patrick not to be fair, and he no longer even had the privilege of being the youngest of the household.

Teenagers often seem particularly ill at ease if their mother or father develops a new relationship which shows signs of being permanent, and can become very difficult with the 'intruder'. They are beyond the younger child's state of wanting a new mummy or daddy at home, but are not yet mature enough to share their parent or allow them to become fully involved in a new love relationship – after all surely they are too old for that! This may also be a time when they begin to take responsibility for visiting or even seeking out their own 'missing parent', and may unrealistically begin to think that life would be better if they changed families. Sadly, difficult teenagers are not easily welcomed into their other parent's home or new family, and sometimes repeated breakdowns of relationships occur and the youngster may end up homeless or in care.

Yet, despite all this gloom, many second marriages are successful, and many families have begun to learn the art of coping with the often complex sets of relationships implied by the term 'step'.

It is helpful to bear in mind that most children would really like to have an ideal mum and dad, together always. If this breaks down then they need some explanation at the time and then further explanations as they grow older. Children may wish to keep the possibility of a reunion open, and so initially resist a new arrival in the household.

The new husband or boyfriend may be accepted straightforwardly as 'Dad' or 'my second dad' or by their first name – 'Uncle' seems to have gone out of fashion. These different names do not happen by accident and are likely to reflect something about the agreed role of the man in the household. There are no absolute rights and wrongs to this.

Remember that your children are probably also trying to protect you and want you to be happy – sometimes the way they show this is hard to fathom. Don't imagine that a new happy standard family can be easily and instantly created. The children will be thinking about the paren

hey are no longer with and with whom they will want to
ave contact. Swallow your pride and try to make this
ossible in as peaceful a way as possible. Many families
re quite proud of the complex series of half- and step-
elatives they have, and keep in contact with the wider
amilies at festivals and birthdays. This can often come in
seful if there is a crisis, say over child-minding or if a teen-
ger needs a temporary break from his or her own family.

Because so many family networks now have experience
f divorce and remarriage there is less of a stigma and
arents can share their experiences with friends or self-
elp groups. If really tense relationships develop, or one of
he children becomes obviously disturbed, then it is worth
eeking professional help.

Useful organisations

The National Stepfamily Association
  72 Willesden Lane
  London NW6 7TA
  Tel: 081 372 0844 (office): 071 372 0846 (counselling
  service)
rovides support, advice and information for all members
f step-families.

FOSTER AND ADOPTIVE PARENTS

Fostering

ostering was originally arranged mainly by the 'real'
arents who asked someone else to look after their child if
hey themselves were unable do so. It was reasonably clear
vho would make the day-to-day decisions (the foster
arents) and who could decide to end the arrangement
either the foster parents or the real parents). Such an
rrangement could be fairly informal, with relatives or

neighbours, or might involve payment. While this type of more-or-less temporary set-up still occurs, the greatest number of foster placements these days are made by social services trying to provide a family life for children who otherwise would have to be with very unsatisfactory parents or in institutions.

Foster parents, therefore, may have quite a number of other people almost competing with them for the role of parent: first, there may be the child's own 'real', 'first' or 'birth' parents. Second, there is likely to be a social services social worker. And third, there may be some court involvement – for instance if the child is a ward of court. This sort of situation leads to considerable complexities that ordinary parents do not have to face, such as obtaining permission for the child to have medical treatment.

A good 'professional' foster parent may be seen as someone who can take on children at short notice, promote contact with the real parents if appropriate, love and care for a disturbed child, and then give up the child to others after an unpredictable length of time. Emotionally and practically this is a very tall order, and we are lucky that people come forward who are pleased to give children a home for a while.

Long-term fostering – though at one time compared unfavourably with adoption – is now being recognised as having benefits for the child. It can be particularly useful if the foster parents are related to one of the parents, who may be prevented by illness from caring for their own child. Then both child and foster parents can maintain some idea of a positive image about, say, the mother, which will not conflict with allowing love and respect for the foster parents.

Fostering breakdown, however, is unfortunately not uncommon and is upsetting for the children and the adults involved.

Jill, 14, came to the attention of the hospital department because she had taken an overdose of eight
paracetamol tablets. She had been taken into care at the
age of five because of repeated severe beatings from her
father. Her mother, who was mentally and to some
extent physically handicapped, had been unable to
protect her daughter effectively and indeed one younger
child suffered a cot-death.

An aunt offered to take Jill, and social services supervised this as a formal fostering arrangement for a child
who remained in care. Although there were conflicts
within this family Jill did very well – until the aunt
became pregnant and had a row with Jill in which she
hit her. Although Jill was not at all injured, she did feel
rejected and the incident must have recalled for her the
earlier hurts she had received.

When her 'placement' was reviewed Jill said she
didn't want to stay with her aunt any longer and was
removed.

◆

Angus and Sean, aged 11 and 13, were being fostered
by an unrelated couple with no children of their own.
This had been quite a successful arrangement for two
years, but as the children grew older they became
increasingly defiant towards their foster parents and
were very difficult to manage. There seemed to be
pressure on the foster parents to decide whether they
wanted to adopt the children and indeed to 'make them
an offer' to do so. That this would be important
symbolically was evident by everybody's different and
strong feelings about it.

The foster parents felt that Angus (the older boy), in
particular, was too difficult and too involved still with

his mother. The foster mother was extremely fond of the younger boy and certainly wanted to continue to look after him, but adoption seemed like an acknowledgement of her own permanent infertility. The boys loved and hated each other, like most brothers, and still seemed a little ill at ease with the greater wealth and 'poshness' of their new family. Talking about their feelings was a form of torture to them.

In both of these cases, years of loving foster parent input were being put in jeopardy as the children became more challenging as they entered adolescence. It is worth making the point that children who are removed from their parents after neglect or abuse are likely to bear the emotional scars of this and display any of the symptoms that other unhappy and disturbed children do. Because these signs of emotional distress are understandable it does not mean either that they are easy for the caring adults to cope with, or that skilled help and advice cannot be helpful.

The other major feature of the cases above is that the role of the foster parent as *parent* was unclear because it was open to considerable official scrutiny and control. In the end this can be undermining as a child, especially a disturbed one, will always be tempted to push a little bit further to test a parent's commitment if he or she is uncertain of it.

It is not easy for social workers, who are trying to support foster parents, protect the best interests of the child and sometimes also trying to maintain contact with birth parents. If you are a foster parent with a difficult child, do make the best use of the social worker and try to consult with others who have experience of similar situations – whether other parents or professionals.

Remember that fostered children are just as entitled as

others to be referred to child guidance and child psychiatry clinics. Indeed they may be particularly good candidates for child psychotherapy as their most severe environmental problems lie in the past. Thinking of their future mental health, it is obviously crucial to give help while they are young to reduce the likelihood of their becoming caught up in a vicious circle and abusing their own children.

Family advice, sometimes in conjunction with the involved social worker, can also be very helpful in clarifying issues of control and decision-making. Keep in mind that, as well as immediate love and care, if you want children to feel secure and have the best chance of a good emotional development, they need as much of a continuing relationship as possible and to feel that they can rely upon their carers.

ADOPTION

Until fairly recently most children born out of marriage were adopted, and adoptive parents were often middle-class and childless themselves. Now the picture has changed: young single mothers usually choose to bring up their healthy babies themselves and would-be adoptive parents are more likely to be offered older children, or children with some physical or mental handicap.

Adoption is nevertheless usually very rewarding for both parents and children. Once the legal side of the adoption process has been completed there is the security for the child of being brought up in an ordinary family, and no competition with the real parents which is a problem that faces foster parents. Research has shown that children with physical, mental and emotional handicaps who would not previously have been thought suitable for adoption can do extremely well. Of course it is important that the adoptive parents go into this with their eyes open as such children can be demanding and vulnerable.

If you do adopt a young baby the process of emotional attachment is naturally much easier. But family issues you may have to face and resolve include coming to terms with infertility, involving the wider family – such as grand-parents – and of course when and how to tell the child of its origins. Young children are usually quite happy with the idea that they are specially chosen, although they may like to fantasise idealistically about their 'real' parents. Then, as teenagers' identity and origins do become an important focus, a search for the real parents may eventually be undertaken. All of this is quite normal and does not usually threaten the strong bond with the adoptive parents.

If your adopted child does become emotionally disturbed, however, you are bound to feel, even if this feeling is quickly suppressed by guilt, that there could be 'bad blood' or that if the worst came to the worst the child could go back. You don't have to be super-human just because you are an adopter – ask for help.

Children adopted after babyhood are more likely to be emotionally disturbed because of their earlier experiences. Often being with dedicated adoptive parents overcomes this and is one of the reasons why social services frequently look for experienced parents as adopters. However, some children are released for adoption because of very serious abuse and this may be a cause of marked and continued emotional and behavioural disturbance.

Harry, aged six, had been adopted when he was two having been in voluntary care for most of his life while his mother was under psychiatric treatment. The major problem for Harry's adoptive parents was managing his extremely difficult behaviour. He had frequent un-controllable temper tantrums, apparently set off by the slightest frustration of his wishes.

The parents found it difficult to be firm and consistent with each other about this. In the attempt to avoid blaming Harry, who they were only too aware had had a difficult early life, they tended to blame each other or themselves and so added parental quarrelling to the problems.

———————◆———————

Jane took a minor overdose of paracetamol tablets at the age of 14. She was the middle one of three children who had all been adopted and was of mixed racial parentage – unlike her parents. She had begun to feel left out and isolated at school, and when she had a row with a boyfriend she had become very upset. She had also begun to brood about her family of origin but had not felt able to talk about this with her adoptive mother and father. The latter were very shocked and shaken and at one point even began to wonder whether they could cope with Jane any more.

In both of these cases early experiences had probably made the adoptive children vulnerable to psychological disturbance. Another reason for Jane's adolescent identity crisis was having to come to terms with the fact she was from a different racial and cultural origin than her adoptive parents.

The parents found these challenges particularly threatening because the children were adopted. They could not comfort themselves by thinking 'It runs in the family and I was just the same, but I grew out of it'. If one of the parents had been keener on the adoption than the other this can also be a source of marital conflict.

So, if you are an adoptive parent with a difficult child, it is not your fault or theirs. You have undertaken a rewarding but major task and if at some point extra support or psychological treatment seems advisable, do not hesitate to seek it out, and also consider contacting mutual support groups for parents in a similar position.

Useful organisations

Post Adoption Centre
   8 Torriano Mews
   Torriano Avenue
   London NW5 2RZ
   Tel: 071 284 0555
Offers counselling and family work for anyone involved in an adoption.

GAY AND LESBIAN PARENTS

Although gay and lesbian parents may sound like a contradiction in terms, in fact it is not all that uncommon for lesbian and gay people to be in an actual or effective parental relationship with children – with or without a partner. Of course the sexual preference of a member of an openly heterosexual couple may be more complicated than it appears, but this does not usually affect the task of parenthood. However, if such a partnership breaks down and custody of the children is disputed, then the courts have tended to decide in favour of the partner who has acquired a new partner of the opposite sex, and sometimes this factor overrides other issues. Obviously parents, knowing this may happen, may well choose to conceal their inclinations in order to safeguard their relationship with their children.

Nevertheless, there are openly lesbian mothers who look after their children with their partners. If the father has been acknowledged, it may be difficult to maintain continued contact in a positive way. Some women may not have informed the father or may have used artificial aids to conception. There are likely to be difficulties over this for the child at some point, especially if the child is a boy and wants to know more about his father.

Children may also have the usual variety of emotional and behavioural problems, but the caring couple may be reluctant to seek traditional forms of help because they fear criticism of their lifestyle.

Martin, aged eight, was showing very disturbed behaviour in school and so was referred to the child guidance unit. He was brought by his mother and her long-standing female partner who were suspicious of what the clinic might do. In fact Martin's early life had included many disruptions because of the violent breakdown of his parents' marriage, and he had spent time in several children's homes. For his current parents the question was how they could help this little boy to feel more secure.

◆

Polly, aged eight, was the subject of an access dispute being fought by her parents through the court with extreme acrimony. There were accusations and counter-accusations of sexual abuse, almost certainly wildly exaggerated and intended to sway the court in the accuser's direction. The marriage had only fairly recently broken down, and husband and wife had both found new partners with whom they were living – in each case male. The father in fact realised that the court was almost certain to award custody to the mother, and was really trying to establish a reasonable visiting relationship with his daughter, but was finding even this difficult.

Whatever the sexual preference or habits of their parents, children's needs are still the same – for as much secure and continuous affectionate care as possible, and with the least possible family conflict. It is best if they can know, love and respect their real parents and other adults of both sexes. Yet all this is not always possible and many children can grow up reasonably happily under other circumstances. Society and the courts are often unnecessarily disapproving of such arrangements, and that can make it hard for parents to seek help.

If you are in this position and considering you may need therapeutic help, it may be worthwhile 'shopping around' if that is possible. For instance, you might want to find out if a clinic can offer you the possibility of a female therapist, or you might want to find out what their experience is with non-traditional families and their attitudes towards them.

Useful organisations
Lesbian and Gay Switchboard
   BM Switchboard
   London WC1
   Tel: 071 837 7324
Provides 24-hour information and help.

Lesbian Line
   BM Box 1514
   London WC1
   Tel: 071 251 6911
Provides advice, information and help.

PARENTS OF DIFFERENT RACES

When two people from different races marry they are likely to be from different cultures. So on the one hand there may be obvious differences of appearance, especially of skin colour and perhaps of language. On the other hand, more subtle cultural differences such as assumptions about marriage roles, family customs and child-rearing may not even be evident to the couple themselves until later. The first real challenge is usually the potential in-laws, which may lead to a temporary or permanent rift or coolness. The couple's friends may also be more or less approving of the union.

So children of what are called mixed marriages may have to face teasing and prejudice from the outside if their physical appearance makes this obvious, as well as a complex set of relationships with grandparents and other members of the wider family who may have mixed feelings about their very existence. In some localities the situation is fairly common, so there is less of a problem for the child, but in some parts of the country a black or mixed-race child is an oddity and is made to feel such.

Parents of mixed-race children have various problems to face, for instance, what should be the religion adopted for the children? What should be the main language spoken at home?

Although many children come happily through these strains, for some it is an extra stress they cannot cope with.

Josephine, at the age of eight, was noticed by her mother and teacher to be preoccupied with her own skin colour, comparing it unfavourably with whiter-skinned children and favourably with darker-skinned children. Her white English mother was now divorced from her black Afro-Caribbean father and had a new, white partner by whom she had recently had a baby.

Josephine saw her father and his family regularly and even her mother and her partner were on reasonably good terms with them. Yet Josephine was apparently feeling less valued and connecting this with the colour of her skin.

◆

Saul, at 15, was living with both his real parents and was the older of two children. His mother, originally from Jamaica, had a well-paid and responsible job as a senior social worker and his white English father was a teacher. Saul had been doing very well at school until a few months previously when he suddenly started to stay out late and was rude to his parents who suspected he was taking drugs. Saul complained he had always been teased about his colour at school, and was angry with white society. He wanted to explore the company of more black friends and their culture and music. His parents could understand both Saul's wish as an adolescent to explore his cultural connections and even to revolt against their own middle-class values, but were concerned that in his anger at the way society had treated him, Saul might put his whole future at risk.

Parents from different races have probably not been in the position of being of mixed-race themselves and will be learning about the resulting tensions for the family at the same time as the children. Mothers may have to learn different skills of physical care for mixed-race children, and the mother-in-law can usually help with this. Both parents and children may have to learn to cope with insults or rejection, and it will be very important for the children to feel secure and proud of their own identity. Even if one side of the family is taken as the main source of culture and contact, it is helpful for children to know about the other side. As most people will deny any prejudice, this can be a very difficult area to discuss or find information about.

If your child is having emotional problems which may be connected with having a mixed-racial or cultural inheritance, then try to track down a source of help which has some experience of such issues, and which possibly offers special help from people of different ethnic or cultural backgrounds themselves.

Useful organisations

Commission For Racial Equality
    Elliott House
    Allington Street
    London SW1
    Tel: 071 828 7022
Contact the CRE or your local Racial Equality Council for help if your child is experiencing racist trouble at school.

9

WHAT IS TREATMENT LIKE?

To illustrate the kinds of things that happen in assessment and treatment, several cases of encopresis, or soiling, will be described. You will see that an apparently similar problem can have different causes with different children. Treatments may have some things in common, but may also vary – as does the response from the family and the child.

◆

Colin, aged four, attended the hospital clinic with his parents and older sister. He had been referred by a very experienced health visitor who felt she had tried everything without success. The parents received an appointment letter with instructions on how to find the department and asking them to bring the whole family living at home.

When they arrived at the department of child and family psychiatry, which was next to the paediatric outpatients, they checked in with the receptionist and gave some further details. After waiting for a few minutes in the waiting room they were taken down to the interview room by the senior doctor who was going to talk to them.

The interview or observation room was quite large with comfortable chairs, a low table and some toys. What the family particularly noticed were the large mirror on one wall and a video camera. The doctor explained to the parents that she had some colleagues on the other side of the mirror in the next room who could see and hear the assessment, and were there to help. The video was not in use on this occasion.

Colin's mother then began to tell the doctor about the problem. Colin had used the potty and become clean and dry from about 18 months. However, after a hospital admission when he was two he went back to nappies and since then insisted on wearing a nappy to make a poo, even though he used the toilet (sitting or standing) to make a wee. He made a poo at least once a day, sometimes twice; he liked to be by himself, and then have someone to clean him up afterwards.

His parents had tried different methods to get Colin out of nappies – for instance his father said if he made a poo in the toilet he would get a toy car and a party. This was unsuccessful, and indeed when his mother offered Colin the choice of buying nappies or a toy he chose the nappies and seemed very upset by the suggestion of their removal.

Colin was otherwise generally a cheerful and normal little boy, although he did have some anxieties, especially about water. He had only recently begun to accept a bath and hair-wash, and would not go anywhere near the sea.

This anxiety about water clearly dated from the time when, at about two-years-old, he pulled a pan of boiling water over himself. The ambulance men then poured a lot more water over him to cool him down and he was taken to hospital, where his parents were told his chances of living were only 50-50. Luckily he recovered swiftly, but the incident left his mother especially feeling very anxious and protective towards Colin.

The main relevant event in the family history seemed to be that the grandmother on the mother's side had died just before Colin's accident, having been very ill with cancer during the year before.

The older sister of 19, who was still living at home, admitted to worrying a lot about Colin. On the other hand, his father thought that he was less worried than the other members of the family. Colin had a place at nursery but could not go because of the soiling. When his mother thought about him starting school the next year, it 'gave her nightmares'.

Colin played with the toys normally and was prepared to talk a bit and share some of the ideas of his imagination. The doctor thought that Colin, like other children of the same age, might have some fears about the toilet, especially as he was so anxious about water. What was down the toilet? 'Jesus' was the surprising answer. The parents, however, thought they knew what this meant. They had told Colin that the granny who had died had 'gone to live with Jesus', and more recently when the pet goldfish died it had been 'buried' with a little ceremony down the toilet. Colin went on: there could also be a big elephant down the toilet (picked up toy elephant). What could he do? He could get another elephant and hit him (he acted this out with the toys).

'What about the sea – why is that worrying?' asked the doctor. Colin answered 'The water might suck you up and you have to have a boat.'

After talking to each of the family members for about three-quarters-of-an-hour the doctor went into the next room to talk with colleagues, and hear their observations and views.

It was thought that Colin's fears and his reluctance to use the toilet or even the potty to make a poo appeared to date from the traumatic experience of a bad scalding at the age of two. His mother was sensitised anyway by the recent illness and death of her own mother and continued to have many fears for Colin, which were probably reduced by letting him behave like a very protected baby. In fact the family as a whole seemed generally rather anxious and depressed.

The doctor returned to the family in the interview room and advised the parents not to make threats or big offers of rewards and bribes. The most helpful thing until the next appointment would be just to keep a chart showing how often and where Colin was making his poos. It was thought possible Colin might even make some suggestions himself, for instance he might want to use a pot for a while.

Further family meetings were recommended to hear more from Colin about his worries, and why everyone else's anxieties are focused on him.

The next appointment was three weeks later and the interview was in a different room without the mirror. The family – who this time had come without the father – were much more relaxed than on the first occasion. They reported that Colin seemed more confident at home too – but he still insisted on a nappy. The doctor wondered with the mother and sister how long it would be all right for Colin to carry on with his nappies, and whether he could give them up gradually or suddenly. The sister thought the nappies should all be completely thrown out at once. The mother found this idea extremely upsetting because of the fuss Colin had made when an attempt was made to do this once before.

The doctor advised that getting rid of the nappies all

at once was probably a good idea, but would be a considerable challenge. All the adults in the family should agree between themselves when the right moment should be, and the father's involvement in this would be crucial. Obviously it would have to be some time in the next six months as Colin was then due to start school. To encourage Colin, he was given a chart with shiny red stars which he would earn for each poo he made in the toilet. He was quite enthusiastic about this.

The next appointment, for three weeks later, was cancelled by the mother, but she rang the doctor a week later. She had not felt able to stop the nappies at once, but on a convenient day told Colin they had run out and she was not getting any more. He had been first angry then sulky. He did not make a poo at all for the next day and complained of tummy-ache. However, no nappy appeared and he later took himself off to the toilet and was pleased to show a success! Since then he was so proud of himself and the stars he was earning, and there was no further soiling problem. His mother was also rightly quite proud of her own efforts, and was planning to take Colin to nursery school as soon as possible.

Psychiatrist's comments

There are theoretical arguments about whether it is best in therapy with children to concentrate on the symptom or to emphasise helping the child and family to understand their anxieties or to communicate better. If the family does not have too many overwhelming problems, they often respond well to a combination of approaches.

In this case, it was not too difficult to understand why Colin was anxious about water and clung on to some of the habits of a younger child. Just talking gently about what had happened, and letting everybody say something about their fears, probably helped quite a lot. At the second appointment a specific plan of action was suggested by one family member and supported by the doctor with acknowledgement that it would be difficult for a short while. The child was brought into the discussion and the 'behavioural' approach of a star chart was used. However, the decision-making and implementation of the plan was up to the parents, and they succeeded very well. It is interesting that with the success over the toileting, the mother's fears about Colin starting school reduced enormously.

Henry was nearly three when he was seen at the hospital child and family psychiatry department. He had also been referred by a health visitor. Before sending an appointment the psychiatrist rang the health visitor. Soiling was not usually considered a problem at the age of two – was child psychiatry really necessary? The health visitor knew the family very well and thought that the mother and grandmother were desperate for help, and in addition there was another difficulty because Henry did not accept that his great-grandmother had died (a fairly recent event).

As with the preceding case the family – which consisted of Henry with his mother and grandmother – were interviewed by the doctor all together in the observation room.

Both the mother and grandmother told the story: Henry was out of nappies but sometimes 'made his plops' in his pants or on the floor. He sometimes went for days without passing a bowel motion. He preferred the toilet to a potty and did use it appropriately sometimes. There did not seem to be a pattern in time of day

when he passed a motion, but his mother and grandmother could tell when he was about to as he sat on the
floor with his knees out and went quiet.

The mother and grandmother wanted Henry to stop
soiling so that he could start nursery school. They said
they had tried 'everything' – but in fact this turned out
to be only negative things such as smacking and telling
off.

The grandmother had started to 'train' Henry from
six weeks, and did get him 'clean and dry' by 18
months. She had done the same thing successfully with
her own three children. Henry's later relapse into
soiling was not thought to be related to any particular
events or stresses. Laxatives were tried once but did not
seem to help. The mother linked the constipation
symptoms with her own experience of constipation,
which had got much worse after Henry's birth.

Henry was described as having been insecure, for
instance wanting to cuddle, not liking being left at
playgroup and waking up frightened, but this had
improved recently. He was a 'great charmer' especially
with adults, but was not yet very friendly with other
children.

Henry's birth and early development were normal.
His parents had quarrelled at his birth and the father
had not continued contact. His mother returned to live
with her own parents and went back to work. During
the day Henry had been looked after by his great-
grandmother or his grandmother. It emerged that both
the great-grandmother and the grandmother saw Henry
as a 'replacement' for Jack – the grandmother's
younger brother who had tragically died at the age of
three.

Henry was indeed a charmer. At first he was shy
with the interviewer, but he became quite chatty later.

His speech was very good, with many adult turns of phrase. He enjoyed playing with the tea-set and then the fire engine.

The adults were fairly subdued, and insisted that they had no disagreements about Henry's upbringing. Potentially difficult areas such as Henry's father, the mother's current boyfriend and Henry's future pattern of care seemed to be avoided. The grandmother in particular seemed hopeless about the likely outcome and was quite critical of her daughter and her grandson; she could not accept that occasional soiling at the age of two was acceptable or normal.

After about 50 minutes the interviewer went into the next room to consult with the observers, who, on this occasion, were a child psychotherapist and two medical students.

It was agreed that Henry was an advanced little boy for his age in most respects, and that this precocity might have contributed to his grandmother's not realising that toilet lapses and not understanding death are quite normal with little children. It was also thought it would be useful to spend more time on a future occasion asking more about the different members of the family in order to understand more about the relationships.

This discussion was fed back to the family by the psychiatrist and they were given a star chart to use with Henry, who would earn a star every time he made a poo in the toilet.

At the second session, grandmother, mother and Henry again met with the child psychiatrist. They had brought along the star chart which showed that Henry had earned five stars for making poos in the toilet and there had been no major soiling at all. Interestingly, it was when the mother's boyfriend was with him that

Henry asked to go to the toilet for the first time.

Both mother and grandmother expressed concerns that he might be experiencing some pain. They related the difficulty to the mother's own experience; following a tear from Henry's birth, she had to have a 'stretch' because of pain, bleeding and constipation. It was suggested that there was probably a vicious circle of withholding and hardness of the poos, so that using a laxative occasionally was very sensible. If this continued to be a problem we would ask advice from a paediatrician. Henry was very pleased about his stars and cheerfully drew a picture of a poo.

Everyone seemed much more relaxed; mother was more forthcoming and grandmother less critical. They told the therapist more about the way they shared Henry's care and about mother's boyfriend, who was a regular visitor and well-liked by Henry who sometimes called him 'Dad'. Henry didn't know anything about his own real father, but when he does ask, he will be told the truth.

Grandmother commented that what with Henry being tall and generally advanced he was often expected to behave in ways beyond his years, but none of her three children had soiled beyond the age of 18 months. Henry had not yet given up the idea of his great-grandmother being still in hospital rather than dead, and the therapist suggested that he did seem to 'hold onto' some things such as poos and ideas.

The advice was to carry on with the chart which was going well. The third session took place a month later, again with Henry, mother and grandmother. Excellent charts were produced. There had been no soiling at all, and Henry had gained extra stars when he asked to go to the toilet without being prompted.

Mother, grandmother and Henry were all very

pleased and thought that there were now no other problems. In fact they thought Henry had made good progress all round. Grandmother mentioned the great-grandmother's death again. This time, however, she said that although Henry insisted she was still in hospital perhaps this was a nice way of holding onto her memory, and that he would realise in his own time what had happened.

As such good progress had been made the family were not offered a further fixed appointment, but could make contact at any time in the future if they wished.

Psychiatrist's comment

At first this child's symptoms did not sound as if they needed treatment, yet in fact because of the level of family distress an intervention was well worthwhile. Most children's problems arise from number of factors coming together, which is why it is helpful to obtain full details of recent family stresses and conflicts, as well as a developmental history of the child. It is not all that unusual to find that one of the relevant events happened many years ago, but still has a great deal of importance to family members. In this case, it was the childhood death of a great-uncle.

At the end of the first session a star chart was given. Note the emphasis is always on simple rewards for clear and agreed actions. When the problem is soiling 'being clean' is not a specially desirable outcome, as this target can lead to the child becoming constipated in the effort to earn stars, so 'poos in the toilet' is a better aim. Physical issues have to be considered, but do not always need complex medical help.

There seemed to be an all round improvement with clear reduction of family stress and mutual criticism. These issues were not addressed directly, but were probably aided by allowing the family to speak in their own way about the loss of the great-grandmother, the way the two women shared Henry's care, and their thoughts about the role of a father in Henry's life.

Kevin, who was nearly six, was referred by his GP and came with his mother to the appointment at the hospital child psychiatry clinic. They were seen together by the child psychiatrist.

His mother told how Kevin had a pattern of not passing any bowel motions for up to two weeks. Then with or without laxatives he passed 'small bits', mostly in his pants, and sometimes in the toilet. The reaction from his parents varied from time to time, but both his mother and his father had got angry and smacked him.

The mother thought that Kevin had a fear and dislike of the toilet and recounted that he had fallen in twice when younger which could account for this. There was no problem of wetting.

The pattern of constipation needing laxatives had been present since Kevin was two weeks old, but had been checked out twice by the hospital paediatricians who said there was no physical problem and that he would grow out of it.

Apart from the early history of constipation Kevin's development had been quite normal, and he had been looked after at home by his mother until he started school. Kevin was getting on quite well at school, which he enjoyed, although he sometimes had to be kept off to get his bowels 'sorted out'.

Kevin was the only child. His parents had both been born in London and were from supportive families of Afro-Caribbean origin. The father had had similar problems to Kevin as a child, but did not like to talk about them. The mother was expecting another baby in about two months.

Kevin was a well-built little boy, who drew quietly at first but then became very responsive. He indicated by his facial expression that he didn't like the toilet, or making a poo, but that a potty was not so bad. He drew a tiger, which 'lives in the jungle and has big claws – to kill people with'. He liked to go out with his father to play football in the park. He thought it would be nice to be 'fixed' one day and be happier about pooing and toilets. Mother was rather quietly spoken, but her remarks about Kevin were predominantly critical.

The initial impression was that Kevin had a long-standing problem of soiling associated originally with constipation, and now also with withholding and fearful avoidance of the toilet. He had probably been brought for help at this point because another baby was on the way.

Further appointments were offered to concentrate on reducing the symptom of soiling; the mother was asked to encourage the father to attend if possible. The initial suggestions were:

- The parents were to avoid criticism as much as possible for the time being.
- Mother was to keep a chart of the type and place of bowel movements.
- Kevin was to choose a potty with his mother that he would enjoy using for a 'training period' before going on to the toilet.

Kevin was enthused by this and said 'Sounds good to me!' – so off they went.

At the second appointment a week later mother and Kevin attended. Kevin was very pleased about the potty he had chosen, had used it once and been 'clean' since.

The mother had kept a conscientious record.

Kevin chatted about his fears about the toilet: 'There are giant rats and snakes down there ... in the sea'. What could Kevin do about this? 'I would stab them all to death with a knife and fly back in an aeroplane.... It's not safe yet ...'

It was agreed to amend the programme so that Kevin would get a silver star to be traded in for five pence for each time he made a poo in the potty.

At the third session three weeks later another excellent chart was produced. Kevin was making poos in the potty two or three times a week (for 10 pence!) and had no dirty pants. His mother said he seemed to want to be nagged and Kevin agreed; he did not want to use the toilet yet. Mother was amazed and very pleased by the good progress, so as they seemed to be winning they were advised to continue.

The family missed the next appointment, so were followed up by phone two months later. Mother reported that Kevin was now using the toilet successfully, and she had just produced a baby girl. Kevin claimed to be 'not quite OK' – he wanted to come back to the clinic again.

Psychiatrist's comment

With Kevin the main issue was soiling and fear of the toilet arising originally from constipation and also having fallen in. This had probably been made worse by the parents' understandable resulting irritation and criticism. It was interesting that the father had a similar problem as a child, about which he did not like to speak (or presumably think), which made helping his own son difficult. Although it would have been useful to have the father along too, the mother was able to follow through with the advice herself and certainly the little boy was keen to make progress at his own pace.

Again, the simple star chart was successful. This time a 'trade-in' value (not too high) was attached as over-fives understand and respond well to this. Kevin's fears were also explored and accepted – a process which he clearly found very reassuring in itself. It was also probably an important time in Kevin's life to ensure that he felt loved and appreciated, as he was about to be faced with a new small rival.

◆

Simon, aged nine, was brought to the hospital clinic by his mother following referral from the school nurse. His mother brought him with his younger brother, and they all seemed rather anxious about the interviewing room with its mirror and camera. However, the mother agreed to proceed when given an explanation about its purpose.

The problem was once again soiling, and also extreme shyness at school. Simon and his mother did not seem to have the right words to describe the difficulty, but eventually agreed on 'not doing toilet in the toilet'. It turned out that Simon sometimes soiled his pants and never used a grown-up toilet, only a potty.

Simon only spoke in monosyllables throughout the interview, turning to his mother to answer when he was asked questions. The little brother was also very restrained for a small child.

It turned out that Simon had had an extremely difficult start to life; he was born premature and then had to have several heart operations, which created a great deal of anxiety for his parents. At first he seemed to be delayed in his development, especially in speech, but when he started school he did surprisingly well academically. However, he hardly spoke at all to the other children, though he did not seem to be bullied. He did not play outside much, but drew and wrote a lot at home, making up his own comic strips.

The soiling had only been occurring for a few months and was possibly related in time to an admission for yet another hospital operation – this time the bringing down of an undescended testicle. Simon's mother also thought that he had been upset when he had to go up into the main school from the infants – a period that coincided with the death of her mother and also with the birth of the little brother Paul.

Simon's mother did not seem to be someone who would respond angrily to soiling, but she did seem very anxious about her son and this was understandable given the difficult start in life he had had. Despite that, he was in some ways doing very well.

The team watching the interview were struck by the quietness, even sadness of the family, and it did seem likely that there was more to learn. The interviewer asked the mother to bring along the father the next week.

At the second interview the mother, father and both children attended. Although they all still seemed a bit shy, the feeling of great anxiety and unhappiness seemed to have diminished. Both children began to play appropriately, even though Simon would still not say much. Simon's father agreed about the main problems – soiling and shyness especially at school.

First the soiling and use of the potty was discussed. The interviewer wondered at what age the father thought it appropriate for his son to stop using the potty – at 10, perhaps at 12? 'Today' the father said firmly. The interviewer thought that a nine-year-old boy definitely needed his father to show him the right way to use the toilet – man to man – and that this was something that a mother might not be able to do. Everybody seemed quite happy with this suggestion, and ways to help Simon get out more to play were also discussed.

The father did not attend the third session, but mother and the two children did. Toileting was no longer a problem; instead mother was now primarily concerned about Simon's reluctance to speak in public and how he could possibly manage in secondary school – which now seemed to be approaching fast. She wondered if early speech therapy could have caused the problem, but this seemed unlikely. Again, Simon seemed quite relaxed in drawing and playing but would not answer questions requiring more than a 'yes' or a 'no'. Instead he would make a non-committal 'mm?' and turn to his mother as if she should reply.

It was clear that a new and more difficult symptom had emerged which was likely to need a different therapeutic approach and would probably take quite a long time to improve. Simon's mother was keen on the idea of individual therapy for Simon and it was agreed that the next step would be to arrange this. As the family left the room, the mother suddenly said 'Could the death of a baby cause this? When Simon was four-years-old I had another little boy who also had heart problems, and he died at a few months old. He would be just starting school now.'

The next phase of treatment was then entered into; Simon was seen weekly by a child psychotherapist to help him explore and resolve his anxieties, and the parents were offered appointments at the same time by a psychiatric social worker to discuss the difficulties with Simon and also consider the influences in their own lives which were contributing to the situation.

Psychiatrist's comment

Simon's soiling problem was of a fairly recent onset and resolved fairly quickly once the family had been brought together to consider how to sort it out. However, its resolution did not improve Simon's other long-standing difficulties of adjustment – instead it highlighted how important further help was. Simon could in fact be described as an elective mute, that is to say he could speak perfectly well (at home), but refused to do so in other places (school and hospital).

It is quite common in child psychiatric treatment to find that there is a shift of 'goal', sometimes if the original symptom improves as in this case, and sometimes even if it doesn't.

———————— ◆ ————————

Alan was referred again to the department by his GP at the age of 12. He had been seen before when younger and received a lot of help for similar symptoms of soiling, wetting and starting fires, which had largely resolved previously but now re-emerged. In addition he was now misbehaving in school and failing to make much educational progress.

The family were first seen together by a child psychiatrist and a psychiatric social worker, as it was obviously a complex and long-standing case. The previous therapists had left but there were good records at the clinic, so the parents did not have to explain the story all over again.

Alan was the only boy and the youngest of three children; he was very evidently immature in many ways as well as being the baby of the family – and the symptoms of soiling and wetting, appropriate for a younger child, served to underline this.

Looking back at Alan's life with the parents, it

seemed that the extent of his symptoms related closely to his mother's state of health. For instance, she had been so depressed after his birth that she had been admitted to hospital. During the time previously that she had been seen at the department on a weekly basis by a psychiatric social worker things had considerably improved. During the year of the re-referral the mother had developed a severe form of epilepsy and had collapsed several times in front of Alan looking as if she was dead.

Near the end of the first interview the two therapists left the room to discuss the case together. They thought that the parents, probably through anxiety and lack of confidence, found it difficult to present Alan with the firm and consistent guidelines he needed. Alan also had very real problems of his own which needed further investigation.

It was then put to the family that regular sessions of family therapy would be offered to help the parents manage Alan's severe difficulties. Alan was also referred to a paediatrician to check if there were any physical reasons for his wetting and soiling. The school was also asked to make an assessment of Alan as it seemed likely he had special educational needs.

The family attended regularly over the next few months, but things seemed to get worse rather than better. The parents had found even keeping a simple chart difficult, and nothing seemed to be happening by way of assessment or extra support at school. The paediatric investigation had found no underlying physical causes for Alan's symptoms.

At the next family meeting the possibility of individual child psychotherapy for Alan was offered and accepted, and an assessment of his learning capabilities by a clinical psychologist was arranged.

Alan then started to attend for regular weekly sessions with a child psychotherapist in the department, which lasted for about a year. Meanwhile his parents were seen together fortnightly by the child psychiatrist and the psychiatric social worker.

The clinical psychologist reported that while Alan had other average skills, he had very great difficulties with words. This meant that, for instance, reading and writing were very difficult for him, though some other tasks he could perform quite well. This sort of situation was bound to lead at school to remarks such as 'could do better', and Alan was the kind of boy who would probably try and cover up his inadequacies by pretending that he wouldn't rather than couldn't do his school work.

The parents found that in sessions without Alan it was easier to work out how they could best help him, and Alan also benefited from his individual therapy sessions so that the symptoms at home abated. Although there were considerable delays, eventually the school responded to the promptings of the parents and the hospital and provided Alan with some additional educational support, but progress there remained slow and uncertain.

Psychiatrist's comments

Alan's symptom of soiling was one of many, indicating a severe disturbance. Although he had previous considerable therapeutic help his problems had re-emerged under stress and it became increasingly clear that he was a very vulnerable boy who would need a lot of help. The skills of all of the different professionals based in the child psychiatric department were needed, and in addition paediatric investigations and educational assessment and help were also required.

10

SELF-HELP GROUPS

Apart from the NHS and private services, another source of help for those coping with a child who is difficult, disabled or ill is the self-help group.

The number of self-help groups have been growing steadily over the last decade. Some have been set up by parents who have looked for a specific kind of help regarding their child, failed to find it and tried to fill the gap themselves by starting a group which offers advice and information about a specific problem, disease or disability.

Take **Stepfamily** (the National Stepfamily Association) for example. Elizabeth Hodder, the founder and co-director, is married with seven children, five of them step-children. She was, therefore, very aware of the difficulties step-children go through and the need for an organisation for step-parents that offered knowledgeable, specific help and counselling. Over six million adults and children in Britain now live in step-families.

Stepfamily consists of a number of associated groups around the country, run by step-parents. At these, step-parents can discuss the problems of their children and their step-children, which they may have difficulty in doing at home because of being overheard.

For example, 13-year-old Anne's mother had left home to live with another man. Anne's father remarried a woman who already had two teenage children. At a group meeting, the father said that Anne continued to regard these children as intruders. And his ex-wife, who left him, was still causing problems, mainly concerned with the fortnightly access. She wouldn't come and pick up the children, and she was always buying clothes and tapes for them and asking them what her father and his new wife argued about. The group suggested they contacted a local family conciliation service, which aims to help couples sort out differences about arrangements for their children through conciliation rather than confrontation.

This particular group also organised a day out together with their children and step-children. It gave members a chance to see the problems experienced by other families which they had previously only heard about. Many of these involve complex relationships, like jealousy between step-children and the other children combined with feelings of guilt.

Listening to members of such a group talking, the stress is evident. It is obviously more helpful to share and defuse this tension among adults who understand the situation than to pass the tension onto your children.

As well as local groups, **Stepfamily** provides telephone counselling. Members can also buy information packs, booklets and books and attend any conferences and seminars organised by the association. They also receive a quarterly newsletter and there is now a children's newsletter, written by step-children for step-children, called *Stepladder*.

Many self-help groups give you an opportunity to contact other parents in the same situation and discuss problems, exchange advice and obtain information.

The **Cry-sis Support Group** is another example of one of the many groups that offers support and advice. It was set up in 1981 and aims to help mothers of babies who cry excessively and/or have sleep problems.

You may have been spending sleepless nights trying to soothe a colicky, unhappy baby and be suffering from an immense amount of stress and tiredness. Your feelings of depression, anger, frustration and exhaustion may even have reached the point when you feel you could harm the baby. The baby's behaviour may strike you as abnormal to the extent that you are losing your confidence as parents, and you may be convinced that no one else can possibly understand your feelings.

You can get help from health visitors, midwives and your GP, but due to pressure of time they may not be able to give the lengthy support that you want. **Cry-sis** provides a life-line. It is mainly a listening and understanding service, run by parents who have gone through the same difficulties and feelings. It also provides much-needed information. When you have a constantly crying baby it is easy to attribute this to your own inadequacy as a parent. If you have become convinced this is the case it can be very comforting, for instance, to be told that some 10 per cent of all babies cry constantly and an even higher percentage have poor sleep patterns.

Cry-sis publishes several newsletters a year. It offers parents practical advice and guidelines on how to cope and reduce their stress based on the experiences of hundreds of parents who have contacted the group. Such suggestions include having regular breaks by leaving the baby with a relative or neighbour, getting out of the home as often as possible and trying to find a sympathetic listener with whom they can share their feelings.

The need for such an organisation has been demonstrated by the way a whole network of groups and contacts has now developed around the country. And although it does not offer medical advice – anyone with a constantly crying child should see their GP or health visitor – **Cry-sis** is one of the many self-help groups that provide sensible advice and help parents psychologically.

Although parents usually turn to their GP first when faced with a problem with their child, self-help groups can be most helpful when a child has a specific or rare disease, because of the accumulated knowledge they can pass on. The **Tay Sachs and Allied Diseases Association** is an example of an organisation that can help you when your child is suffering from a rare disease.

A GP, for instance, may not have detailed knowledge of Tay Sachs disease – an incurable, inherited condition that leads to a progressive deterioration in the nervous system of young infants and death by the time they reach the age of four or so. The Association publishes booklets and dispenses information about the disease. It aims to provide help and support to families of affected children, as well as putting families in touch with each other.

Any illness or problem affecting one child is liable to affect other children in the family as they may resent the attention and time that the ill or problem child is getting. By being able to talk to other parents about how they deal with this you may have fresh ideas on how to cope.

There are other self-help groups who offer specific expertise in other fields. If, for instance, you are worried that your child may be sniffing glue or other solvents, or taking drugs, it is sensible to talk to the relevant self-help organisations so that you can get as much information as possible. Both **Re-Solv**: the Society for the Prevention of Solvent and Volatile Substance Abuse and **Release** (which provides a 24-hour telephone advice and information service dealing with drugs) are the kinds of agency that can help you.

Some groups provide help for both the child as well as the parent. Take gambling. An addiction to fruit machine gambling can have a disastrous effect on both the child teenager and you as the parent, as the need to find money for gambling may result in the child stealing, disobeying or behaving defiantly. This naturally disrupts the family and you can well be at your wits' end trying to deal with your son (it is mainly boys who gamble).

Gamblers Anonymous has over the last few years incorporated many young gamblers addicted to fruit machines. At Gamblers Anonymous group meetings youngsters can talk voluntarily about their lifestyle. Sometimes a social worker or even their GP suggests they go to the group. It is not compulsory for them to stay and, indeed, some go for one session and do not return.

Other youngsters in the group help newcomers, based on their own experiences. For example, at one meeting a young gambler, who had succeeded in giving it up, suggested to those still addicted: 'Stop gambling for just one hour at a time. Say to yourself: "Tonight I'm not going to the arcade." Then try to plan what to do instead, even if it's just washing dishes in a restaurant.' Another said that stopping gambling wasn't enough: 'You have to fill the void that it leaves. It's a good idea to take up sport or some kind of hobby.'

These groups are often successful because young people are much more likely to take advice from contemporaries, rather than from you.

Gam-Anon, which is an offshoot of Gamblers Anonymous, focuses on the relatives of compulsive gamblers and, through literature and self-help groups, helps them in a similar way to Gamblers Anonymous. Groups for the compulsive gambler are held in the same building so that all members of the family, if they so wish can be helped simultaneously.

Alateen, an offshoot of Alcoholics Anonymous and run on similar lines, gives support and understanding to teenagers who are, or who have been, affected by an alcoholic parent. At group meetings, teenagers have the chance of being quite open about their feelings, knowing that those listening are not going to be patronising as they have suffered from exactly the same problem. If their feelings are not aired, there could be a serious build-up of stress which could have explosive results. What is often surprising at these groups is the humour teenagers show in describing the situations in which they have found themselves. This, and shared feelings, play a considerable part in reducing stress all round.

Some groups offer a telephone helpline which can help you if you are in particular distress. Some crises arise that require instant help at an impossible time like late on a Sunday night. Certain organisations run telephone helplines or lifelines which can at least take the immediate heat out of the situation. These are run by volunteers who have faced similar problems themselves and can offer advice.

An example is **Parents' Anonymous Lifeline** which is a strictly confidential telephone service available to anyone who is having problems with their babies, toddlers or older children. By being able to talk to someone who understands what you are going through, you may be saved from striking a child or behaving in some way that will make reconciliation with an older child very difficult.

It may be that the crisis you are facing is not caused by your child's behaviour but because of your child's serious illness. This is particularly hard to bear and your reaction and the amount of time spent visiting the sick child could understandably have an effect on any other children in the family.

If your child is seriously ill, you will need help over this short-term crisis. But many of you may be facing what is, in effect, a long-term crisis – when your child is physically or mentally handicapped. A number of organisations provide help in these circumstances, like **Contact a**

'amily. This is a parents' telephone service which puts
amilies who have physically and/or mentally handi-
apped children in touch with each other, so that they are
ble to give each other support and practical help, as well
s the opportunity to share information.

The advantage of these voluntary groups is therefore
hreefold: they can provide information about the specific
roblem or difficulty, practical advice and, above all, they
an give you help and support if you have been coping
lone with a particular situation and feel totally isolated.
'or example, you may not want to confide in your rela-
ives or neighbours if your child is taking drugs or is a
ompulsive fruit machine gambler or is slowly dying from
 disease. But if you have a chance to meet or talk to
thers in a similar situation, who genuinely understand
xactly what you and the rest of the family are going
hrough, it can be of inestimable psychological help.

The **Eating Disorders Association** is another organis-
tion which holds self-help groups to which the anorexic
r bulimic and you as a parent are invited. (It may be more
ppropriate with younger sufferers, however, to offer them
ndividual help and the EDA may be able to suggest
omeone in your local area who can help.)

Anorexics tend to be very secretive. Self-help groups
ffer them the chance to talk about their situation publicly
vith other anorexics, discuss the causes of the condition
vith the group, and give themselves individual goals to
chieve before the next group meeting. Eighteen-year-old
ylvia, for instance, had bran for breakfast, never had any
unch and went hungry through to supper. She felt guilty
t even having supper and cut this to a minimum, going
vithout it altogether every third day. The group leader
uggested she gave herself the goal of having something to
at at lunchtime, even if it was no more than a token meal.
he encouraged Sylvia not to feel guilty at this, or go

without supper because she had eaten a minimal amount at lunch. She asked Sylvia to think whether she really did want to get better: if she was sincere about it, then she would have to try to re-establish a normal eating pattern.

Families of anorexics also need help; and the **Eating Disorders Association** can offer help, support and understanding by phone and post. Over the years it has built up a comprehensive amount of information about anorexia and bulimia nervosa which it is willing to pass on.

Voluntary associations are not a replacement for possible psychological or psychiatric treatment, but they are excellent in dispensing information and defusing stress.

Addresses of relevant groups are listed in the address section at the back of the book.

11

HOW TO GET THE BEST RESULT

Whether you are at the stage of thinking about getting help for your child's emotional problems, or assessment and treatment have actually begun, or you have already contacted a self-help group, there are things that you, as parents, can do to help the process along.

Try and think out first what you would like to achieve from the possible service. This might be:

- Knowing more, such as whether your child's behaviour is fairly normal, or whether a pain might have a psychological explanation or a certain behaviour a physical explanation.
- Wanting to understand more, such as how a child's anxieties may be connected up with things that have been stressful for the family in the past.
- Changing the situation, such as lessening family tension or bad behaviour.

You may not know exactly what kind of help you want, but do think about what and how much your family can do to improve the situation. You can then make this clear to the person who is referring the child to the clinic. For example, is everybody in the family willing to attend for the first assessment – in working or school hours? If family treatment is offered is everyone prepared to attend a few times? On many occasions? If individual treatment is offered to the child, are you prepared to accompany him or her and possibly receive parallel therapy? What if the treatment for the child is offered every week, or more often, and may take many months? Sorting out this kind of thing in advance can save a lot of misunderstanding later.

Assessment and therapy sometimes involve reviving uncomfortable, even painful, thoughts and memories. Take things at your own pace if you need to, and remember that the therapists are there to support you and to try to understand. If you cry that is OK, and if your child has a terrible screaming tantrum that's been seen before too.

Sometimes you may be surprised – even made angry – by things that the therapists suggest may have contributed to the problem, or that you should do to help put things right. Of course it is possible that you and the therapist you have met are just ill-matched, but it may be worth your while giving them the benefit of the doubt for a time. After all, whatever you were doing before was presumably not working, and children's problems are often very complex in origin.

Maybe at first you want the therapist to try to control your child or get your errant partner to behave – and perhaps fail as you have! Then at least you feel vindicated. These are understandable wishes, but in the longer run it will be more useful if you yourself gain the confidence to achieve these goals.

Maybe the advice doesn't seem to work completely at first, but consider if nevertheless some parts of it are helpful, or whether there are other difficulties that make the advice impossible to follow and discuss this with the therapist. If you feel cross or anxious or can't understand the reason for something, then do say so. Professionals naturally forget that what is an everyday experience for them is unfamiliar to their clients.

On the other hand, if you find that some advice or discussion or approach is particularly helpful then let the therapist know this too. He or she is not a mind reader and it will guide them in their work with you and also with others. This can be especially helpful when reviewing progress at the end of treatment, as by thinking this through you may learn to manage yourself if a similar problem crops up again.

Remember, you and the therapists have a common aim – the well-being of your child and family. And don't despair about your child; mostly time and nature are on your side.

USEFUL ADDRESSES

Action for Sick Children (National Association for the Welfare of Children in Hospital)
Argyle House, 29–31 Euston Road, London NW1 2SD
Tel: 071 833 2041
Advises families and campaigns for improved standards of care for children in hospital.

Adfam National
1st Floor, Chapel House, 18 Hatton Place,
London EC1N 8ND
Tel: 071 405 3923
National telephone helpline for the families and friends of drug users.

Advisory Centre For Education (ACE) Ltd
IB Aberdeen Studios, 22–24 Highbury Grove, London
N5 2EA
Tel: 071 354 8321
Independent national education watchdog body. Publishes bulletin and gives free advice and support to parents of children in state schools.

Alanon
61 Great Dover Street, London SE1 4YF
Tel: 071 403 0888
Self-help groups for teenagers with alcoholic relatives.

Anything Left-Handed Ltd
   57 Brewer Street, London W1R 3FB
   Tel: 071 437 3910
Distributes items designed for the left-handed.

Association for all Speech Impaired Children
   347 Central Markets, Smithfield, London EC1 A9NH
   Tel: 071 236 6487/3632
Provides support and advice through a network of regional groups; organises conferences, workshops and training for parents and activity weeks for children.

Association for Stammerers
   St Margaret's House, 21 Old Ford Road, London E2 9PL
   Tel: 081 983 1003
Helps and advises those suffering from stammering.

British Diabetic Association
   10 Queen Anne Street, London W1M OBD
   Tel: 071 323 1531
Provides practical help and advice.

British Dyslexia Association
   98 London Road, Reading, Berkshire RG1 5AU
   Tel: 0734 668271
Provides information and the address of your local association.

British Epilepsy Association
   Anstey House, 40 Hanover Square, Leeds LS3 1BE
   Tel: 0532 439393
Provides practical advice and support.

Child Guidance Centres/Clinics
   Details of your local clinic can be found in the phone directory or from the library or the Citizens' Advice Bureau.
   They offer help to children with emotional difficulties and their families. Sometimes you can contact them directly to be seen, or go through your GP or school for referral.

Children's Legal Centre
20 Compton Terrace, London N1 2UN
Tel: 071 359 6251

Provides advice and information on all legal matters relating to children and young people.

ChildLine
Tel: 0800 1111
ChildLine, a free phone service, welcomes phone calls and letters from abused children, including those bullied at school. ChildLine will listen, comfort and protect. Their office address is:
Second Floor, Royal Building, Studd Street,
London N1 0QW
Tel: 071 239 1000 (office)

ChildLine Midlands
Ashley House, 331 Haydn Road, Sherwood,
Nottingham NG5 1DG
Tel: 0602 691199 (office)

ChildLine Scotland
33 Stockwell Street, Glasgow G1 4RZ
Tel: 041 552 1123 (office)

Children Need Grandparents
2 Surrey Way, Laindon West, Basildon, Essex SS15 6PS
Tel: 0268 414607

Gives aid, comfort and advice about gaining contact with grandchildren. An 'action sheet' is available, but please send an SAE.

College of Health
St Margaret's House, Old Ford Road, London E2 9PL
Tel: 081 983 1225

Contact for information on children's health problems including a national waiting list service for non-urgent surgery.

Commission For Racial Equality
Elliott House, Allington Street, London SW1
Tel: 071 828 7022
Contact the CRE or your local Racial Equality Council for help if
your child is experiencing discrimination at school.

Compassionate Friends
6 Denmark Street, Bristol BS1 5DQ
Tel: 0272 292778
A group of bereaved parents who offer help and understanding
to other bereaved parents.

Contact a Family
16 Strutton Ground, London SW1P 2HP
Tel: 071 222 2695
A link service for families who have a physically and/or mentally
handicapped child, so they can share help and support.

Cruse (Bereavement Care)
126 Sheen Road, Richmond, Surrey TW9 1UR
Tel: 081 940 4818
Provides bereavement counselling and advice.

Cry-sis Support Group HQ
BM Cry-sis, London WC1N 3XX
Tel: 071 404 5011
Self-help group which supports parents of babies who cry
excessively or have sleep problems.

Cystic Fibrosis Research Trust
Alexandra House, 5 Blyth Road, Bromley, Kent BR1 3RS
Tel: 081 464 7211
Provides explanatory leaflets and has a nationwide network of
self-help groups.

Defining Dyslexia
132 High Street, Ruislip, Middlesex
Tel: 081 950 1033/868 6810
Provides full, free support system to parents and children unable
to cope with stresses caused by learning difficulties.

Down's Syndrome Association
155 Mitcham Road, London SW17 9PG
Tel: 081 682 4001

Gives practical support, advice and information.

Dyslexia Institute
133 Gresham Road, Staines, Middlesex
Tel: 0784 463935

Has a national network of centres and outposts which offer assessments, tuition, teacher training and support.

Eating Disorders Association
Sackville Place, 44 Magdalen Street, Norwich, Norfolk NR3 1JU
Tel: 0603 621414

Offers help, support and understanding nationwide to all those with eating disorders like anorexia and bulimia.

Education Otherwise
36 Kinross Road, Leamington Spa, Warwickshire CV32 7EF
Tel: 0926 886828
School phobia enquiry line: 0304 210997

Advises those who wish to educate their children at home.

Elfrida Rathbone Islington
34 Islington Park Street, London N1 1PX
Tel: 071 359 7443

Provides a range of services for those with moderate learning difficulties, including an under-fives unit.

Epilepsy Association of Scotland
48 Govan Road, Glasgow G51 1JL
Tel: 041 427 4911

Provides help and information: quarterly newsletter and various publications.

Exploring Parenthood
Latimer Education Centre, 194 Freston Road,
London W10 6TT
Tel: 081 960 1678

Advice and counselling for parents.

Families Anonymous
 Room 8, 650 Holloway Road, London N19 3NU
 Tel: 071 281 8889
Provides support for families of those with drug or alcohol problems, or with an eating disorder.

Family Conciliation Scotland
 127 Rose Street South Lane, Edinburgh EH2 4BB
 Tel: 031 220 1610
Advice concerning custody and access.

Families Need Fathers
 BM Families, London WC1N 3XX
 Tel: 081 886 0970
Helps and advises fathers wanting to remain in contact with their family.

Family Service Unit
 207 Old Marylebone Road, London NW1 5QP
 Tel: 071 402 5175
Encourages disadvantaged families to gain some control over their lives.

Family Welfare Association
 501–505 Kingsland Road, London E8 4AU
 Tel: 071 254 6251
Gives practical help to those in need.

Foundation For the Study of Infant Deaths
 35 Belgrave Square, London SW1X 8QB
 Cot death helpline: 071 235 1721
Provides support, advice and information.

Friedreich's Ataxia Group
    Copse Edge. Thursley Road, Elstead, Godalming,
    Surrey GU8 6DJ
    Tel: 0252 702864
Provides a comprehensive welfare service for all members who
suffer from Friedreich's, cerebellar and other ataxia diseases.
Offers counselling, finance, equipment, holidays, education and
employment. Quarterly magazine, and local contacts.

Gam-Anon
    c/o Gamblers Anonymous, PO Box 88, London SW1 0EU
    Tel: 081 741 4181
Support for relatives or friends of compulsive gamblers.

Gifted Children's Information Centre
    21 Hampton Lane, Solihull, West Midlands B91 2QL
    Tel: 021 705 4547
Information on helping gifted children.

Gingerbread
    35 Wellington Street, London WC2 7BN
    Tel: 071 240 0953
Helps and supports lone parent families through a national
network of self-help groups.

Haemophilia Society
    123 Westminster Bridge Road, London SE1 7HR
    Tel: 071 928 2020
Helps and advises those with haemophilia and their relatives.

Helen House Hospice for Children
    37 Leopold Street, Oxford OX4 1QT
    Tel: 0865 728251
Gives respite care to children with a life-threatening disease and
helps with terminal care.

Home-Start Consultancy
2 Salisbury Road, Leicester LE1 7QR
Tel: 0533 554988
Has details of local teams of volunteers in Britain who offer support, friendship and practical advice to parents having difficulties with their young children.

Hyperactive Children's Support Group
71 Whyte Lane, Chichester, Sussex
Tel: 0903 725182
Provides help and information to families with hyperactive children.

Institute of Psychiatry
De Crespigny Park Road, London SE5
Tel: 071 703 5411
Specialist centre for the assessment and treatment of hyperactive children.

International Autistic Research Organisation
49 Orchard Avenue, Shirley,Croydon CRO 7NE
Publishes results of research.

Kids
80 Waynflete Square, London W10 6UD
Tel: 081 969 2817
Works with parents to help children with developmental or learning problems or who have a mental or physical disability.

Lesbian and Gay Switchboard
BM Switchboard, London WC1
Tel: 071 837 7324
Provides 24-hour information and help.

Lesbian Line
BM Box 1514, London WC1
Tel: 071 251 6911
Provides advice, information and help.

Leukaemia Care Society
   14 Kingsfisher Court, Venny Bridge, Pinhoe, Exeter,
   Devon EX4 8JN
   Tel: 0392 64848
Gives information and support.

ME Association
   Stanhope House, High Street, Stanhope-le-Hope,
   Essex
   SS17 OHA
   Tel: 0375 642466
Provides advice and information.

MIND (National Association for Mental Health)
   22 Harley Street, London W1N 2ED
   Tel: 071 637 0741
Information and advice service for problems concerned with
mental health. Branches throughout Britain.

**National Association of Young People's Counselling and
   Advisory Services**
   Magazine Business Centre, 11 Newarke Street, Leicester
   LE1 5SS
   Tel: 0533 558763
Co-ordinates services for young people aged 16–25.

National Asthma Campaign
   Providence House, Providence Place, London N1 ONT
   Tel: 071 226 2260
Provides information and help for those with asthma and their
families.

National Autistic Society
   276 Willesden Lane, London NW2 5RB
   Tel: 081 451 1114
Provides information and education.

National Children's Bureau
   8 Waley Street, London EC1V 7QE
   Tel: 071 278 9441
Information about resources and research about all children's
issues.

National Children's Home Careline
  85 Highbury Park, London N5 1UD
  Careline (London): 081 514 1177
  Careline (Birmingham): 021 456 4560
  Careline (Leeds): 0532 456456
  Careline (Preston): 0772 824006
  Careline (Maidstone): 0622 756677
  Careline (Taunton): 0823 277133
A phone-in service for people with family problems.

National Council For One Parent Families
  255 Kentish Town Road, London NW5 2LX
  Tel: 071 267 1361
Provides information.

National Deaf Children's Society
  45 Hereford Road, London W2 5AH
  Tel: 071 229 9272
Provides a self-help support service.

National Eczema Society
  4 Tavistock Place, London WC1H 9RA
  Tel: 071 388 4097
Provides information and advice for those with eczema and to their families.

National Family Conciliation Council
  Shaftesbury Centre, Percy Street, Rodbourne, Swindon,
  Wiltshire SN2 AZ
  Tel: 0793 514055
The Council has details of all local family conciliation services, which aim to help couples sort out differences about arrangements for their children through conciliation. Some are free, some charge.

National Schizophrenia Fellowship
  28 Castle Street, Kingston-upon-Thames, Surrey KT1 1SS
  Tel: 081 547 3937
Provides advice and operates regional self-help groups for relatives of those with schizophrenia and allied conditions.

National Society for Epilepsy
Chalfont Centre for Epilepsy, Chalfont St Peter,
Buckinghamshire
Tel: 02407 3991
Provides an education service, and maintains a centre for those
with epilepsy.

National Stepfamily Association
72 Willesden Lane, London NW6 7TA
Tel: 071 372 0844 (office); 071 372 0846 (counselling
service)
Provides counselling and advice on setting up self-help groups.

Newpin
Sutherland House, Sutherland Square, London SE17 3EE
Tel: 071 703 5271
Local branches offer support to carers of children by local
mothers who act as befrienders.

Nigel Clare Network Trust
c/o The Alexandra Gordon Agency, PO Box 44, Woking,
Surrey GU21 5TE
Tel: 0483 724907
Self-help group for families caring for life-limited children.

One Plus One Parent Families Strathclyde
39 Hope Street, Glasgow G2 6AE
Tel: 041 221 7150
Information and advice service to one-parent families in
Strathclyde.

Parents Anonymous Lifeline (London)
6 Manor Gardens,London N7 6LA
Tel: 071 263 8918
Confidental telephone service for distressed parents with
problems with their babies, toddlers or older children.

Parent Network
44–46 Caversham Road, London NW5 2DS
Tel: 071 485 8535
Parent support groups, offering a listening ear and new ideas for handling the ups and downs of family life.

Parents to Parents Information Service
Boddington
Tel: 0327 60295
Provides information on adoption services.

Parentline – Opus
Tel: 0268 757077
Runs groups for parents under stress.

Phobic Action
Greater London House, 547–551 High Road, Leytonstone, London E11 4PR
Tel: 081 558 6012
Helplines, drop-in centres and home visiting.

Post-Adoption Centre
Torriano Mews, Torriano Avenue, London NW5 2RZ
Tel: 071 284 0555
Offers counselling and family work for anyone involved in an adoption.

Relate (National Marriage Guidance)
Herbert Gray College, Little Church Street, Rugby, Warwickshire CV21 3AP
Tel: 0788 573241
Branches around the country providing marriage guidance counsellors, many of whom are also trained to do conciliation.

Release (Legal, Emergency and Drugs Service)
388 Old Street, London EC1V 9LT
Tel: 071 729 9904 (office)
Helpline: 071 603 8654
Provides a 24-hour telephone advice and information service for drug-related problems.

Re-Solv (The Society for the Prevention of Solvent and Volatile Substance Abuse)
30A High Street, Stone, Staffordshire ST15 8AW
Tel: 0785 817885
Provides information, literature and videos aimed to prevent deaths from sniffing solvents and gasses.

Richmond Fellowship (for Community Mental Health)
8 Addison Road, London W14 8DL
Tel: 071 603 6373
Provides care for adolescents from 16 years upwards.

Royal Society for Mentally Handicapped Children and Adults (MENCAP)
Mencap National Centre, 123 Golden Lane,
London EC1Y ORT
Tel: 071 454 0454
Tries to improve life for those with learning disabilities and their parents and carers. Offers counselling, advice, training and education through local societies.

SCOSAC (The Standing Committee on Sexually Abused Children)
73 St Charles Square, London W10 6EJ
Tel: 081 960 6376/969 4808
A service that promotes good practice in child sexual abuse work.

Scottish Council for Single Parents
13 Gayfield Square, Edinburgh EH1 3NX
Tel: 031 557 3121

Provides information and advice to single parents.

Scottish Society for Autistic Children
24d Barony Street, Edinburgh EH1 3JT
Tel: 031 557 0474
Provides help and guidance for parents of autistic children.

Sickle Cell Society
    54 Station Road North, London NW10 4UA
    Tel: 081 961 4006
Provides help, information and support to families affected by sickle cell disease through home and hospital visits, plus financial help when necessary.

Spastics Society
    12 Park Crescent, London W1N 4EQ
    Tel: 071 636 5020
Advice and information for parents of children with cerebral palsy. Call free – Cerebral Palsy Helpline – 0800 626216.

Stillbirth and Neonatal Death Society (SANDS)
    28 Portland Place, London W1N 4DE
    Tel: 071 436 5881
Supports parents who have suffered a stillbirth, late pregnancy loss, or whose baby dies before reaching a month in age, through local self-help groups or individual befriending.

Tay Sachs and Allied Diseases Association
    c/o Royal Manchester Children's Hospital, Hospital Road,
    Pendlebury, Manchester M27 1HA
    Tel: 061 794 4696
Supports affected families.

Turning Point
    Bedford Hall, Bedford Road, London W13
    Tel: 081 567 1215
Charity for those with drug, alcohol and mental health problems. Provides telephone counselling, day centres, residential rehabilitation and research.

Weight Watchers (UK)
    Kidwells Park House, Kidwells Park Drive, Maidenhead,
    Berkshire SL6 8YT
Information available on local groups.

Young Minds
> 22 Boston Place, London NW1 6ER
> Tel: 071 724 7262

Promotes and provides information about services in child and family mental health.

Young People's Counselling Service
> Tavistock Centre, 120 Belsize Lane, London NW3 5BA
> Tel: 071 435 7111, extension 2337

Young people can contact this service direct for advice and counselling.

Youth Advisory Service
> Brook Centre, 153A East Street, London SE17 25D
> Tel: 071 708 1234

Gives advice and information directly to young people, especially about family planning.

Youth Clubs UK
> Keswick House, 30 Peacock Lane, Leicester LE1 5NY
> Tel: 0533 629514

Helps young people develop their physical and mental capacities.

FURTHER READING

Maureen Aarons and Tessa Gittens, *A Handbook of Autism*, Routledge, 1991

Glen Austin, *The Parents' Medical Manual*, Robert Erdmann, 1991

Wayne, R. Bartz and Richard Rason, *Help! I've Got a Kid!: a survival guide for parents*, Exley, 1987

Sue Brooks and Richard Newton, *Down's Syndrome* Optima, 1992

Elizabeth Bryan, *Twins, Triplets and More*, Penguin, 1991

Jo Douglas and Naomi Richman, *My Child Won't Sleep*, Penguin, 1984

Gingerbread and the Community Development Centre, *Just Me and the Kids; A Manual for Lone Parents*, Bedford Square Press, 1990

Paul Hauck, *How to Bring up your Child Successfully*, Sheldon Press, 1982

Rowan Hillson, *Diabetes: a young person's guide* Optima, 1988

Elizabeth Hodder, *Stepfamilies Talking*, Optima, 1989

Patricia Holland, *What is a Child?*, Virago, 1991

Peter Hill, *The Anxious Child*, (available free from The Mental Health Foundation, 8 Hallam Street, London W1N 6DH, Tel: 071 580 0145)

Nancy Kohner and Alix Henley, *When a Baby Dies*, Pandora, 1991

Richard Lansdown and Marjorie Walker, *Your Child's Development from Birth to Adolescence*, Frances Lincoln, 1991

Peter Lambley, *How to Survive Anorexia*, Frederick Muller, 1983

Bryan Lask, *Children's Problems*, Optima, 1985

Brenda Lintner, *Living with Teenagers*, Optima, 1991

Fiona Marshall, *Coping Successfully with your Second Baby*, Sheldon Press, 1991

Alice Miller, *Breaking Down the Wall of Silence: to join the waiting child*, Virago, 1991

Desmond Morris, *Babywatching*, Cape, 1991

Louise Ratkin, *Different Mothers: sons and daughters of lesbians talk about their lives*, Cleis Press, Pittsburgh and San Francisco, 1990

Ann Richardson and Jane Ritchie, *Letting Go: dilemmas for parents whose son or daughter has a mental handicap*, Open University Press, 1989

James Robertson, *Young Children in Hospital*, Tavistock Publications, 2nd edition, 1970

Michael Rosen, *Goodies and Daddies: the A-Z guide to fatherhood*, John Murray, 1991

Peter Rowlands, *Saturday Parent*, Allen & Unwin, 1980

Michael Rutter, *Helping Troubled Children*, Penguin, 1975

Michael Rutter, Barbara Maughan, Peter Mortimore and Janet Ouston with Alan Smith, *Fifteen Thousand Hours*, Open Books, 1979

Douglas Ruben, *Bratbusters! Say Goodbye to Tantrums and Disobediences*, Skidmore-Roth, 1991

Linda Sanford, *Strong at the Broken Places: overcoming the trauma of childhood abuse*, Virago, 1991

Harriet Shiff, *The Bereaved Parent*, Souvenir Press, 1977

Jenny Sutcliffe (ed), *Complete Book of Relaxation Techniques*, Headline, 1991

Eric Taylor, *The Hyperactive Child*, Optima, 1985

Welfare of Children and Young People in Hospital, HMSO, 1991

Miriam Wood, *Living with a Hyperactive Child*, Souvenir Press, 1984

INDEX

N.B. All references are to children unless it is otherwise stated.

BAAF
NFCA